CANCER ETIOLOGY, DIAGNOSIS AND TREATMENTS

DOXORUBICIN

BIOSYNTHESIS, CLINICAL USES AND HEALTH IMPLICATIONS

CANCER ETIOLOGY, DIAGNOSIS AND TREATMENTS

Additional books in this series can be found on Nova's website under the Series tab.

Additional e-books in this series can be found on Nova's website under the -book tab.

CANCER ETIOLOGY, DIAGNOSIS AND TREATMENTS

DOXORUBICIN

BIOSYNTHESIS, CLINICAL USES AND HEALTH IMPLICATIONS

MELINDA PACHE
EDITOR

NOVA BIOMEDICAL

New York

For permission to use material from this book please contact us:
Telephone 631-231-7269; Fax 631-231-8175
Web Site: http://www.novapublishers.com

Library of Congress Cataloging-in-Publication Data

Library of Congress Control Number: 2014931125

ISBN: 978-1-63117-233-5

Published by Nova Science Publishers, Inc. † New York

CONTENTS

PREFACE

Doxorubicin is a classical but useful anti-tumor agent. It is used for the treatment of a variety of malignancies including solid tumors and leukemia due to its broad spectrum anti-tumor activity. It also has well known toxic side effects that must be minimized for its successful use clinically. This book discusses intraperitoneal doxorubicin; preclinical characterization of the drug-delivery device DCBeads for transarterial chemoembolization of doxorubicin and nemorubicin; doxorubicin-induced cardiomyopathy; advanced therapies of doxorubicin by carrier of drug delivery system or combined food components; and prevention and management of cariotoxicity.

Chapter 1 – *Background:* Doxorubicin is a cancer chemotherapy agent with a wide spectrum of activity to a variety of cancers. It also has well known toxic side effects that must be minimized for its successful use clinically. A narrow therapeutic window exists for optimal cancer effects combined with a acceptable toxicity.

Materials and Methods: The application of doxorubicin in the prevention and treatment of peritoneal metastases from colorectal, gastric, and ovarian cancer plus peritoneal mesothelioma has been extensively published. Morbidity and mortality assessments have been recorded. High pressure liquid chromatography has been used to determine drug distribution into peritoneal fluid, plasma, normal and cancerous tissues and urine following doxorubicin administration into the peritoneal space. A large volume of chemotherapy solution has been used to widely distribute the drug to peritoneal surfaces.

Results: Intraperitoneal doxorubicin has been studied in a rat model to determine pharmacokinetic parameters in mammals, possible augmentation by hyperthermia and by pressure. Clinical data in patients has established the parameters for safe drug delivery. Pharmacokinetic studies in humans confirm the favorable pharmacology of intraperitoneal drug delivery for peritoneal metastases patients. The treatment of a large number of patients by early postoperative intraperitoneal drug delivery or by hyperthermic intraoperative drug delivery establishes the clinical utility of this route of administration. Clinical studies in patients with sarcoma, appendiceal malignancy, and colorectal cancer have established this drug in combination with other chemotherapy agents as a standard of care.

Conclusions: Doxorubicin shows characteristics favorable for intracavitary administration and toxicity studies suggest that it is well tolerated by the intraperitoneal route after a major surgical procedure. On the basis of pharmacologic and clinical studies, intraperitoneal doxorubicin has become a global standard of care for hyperthermic perioperative chemotherapy for the management of mesothelioma, sarcoma, appendiceal malignancy, and colorectal cancer with peritoneal metastases.

Chapter 2 – Hepatocellular carcinoma (HCC) represents a challenging malignancy of worldwide relevance and it is one of the most common causes of cancer-related death globally. Therapies that offer a high rate of responses in HCC include surgical resection, transplantation and percutaneous ablation. Among the non-curative therapies, transarterial chemoembolization (TACE) is a minimally invasive approach for palliative treatment of liver tumours combining embolization and chemotherapeutic effects and employed as an adjunctive therapy to liver resection or as a bridge to liver transplantation, as well as prior to radiofrequency ablation. Conventional TACE typically involves the injection of chemotherapeutic agents such as doxorubicin (DX), with lipiodol with or without embolic agent, into the branch of the hepatic artery that feeds the tumor lesion.

Being HCCs poorly responsive tumors, new strategies such as the use of novel drug delivery systems capable of a sustained intra-tumoral release of an anticancer agent with minimal host toxicity warrant investigation. Nemorubicin (PNU-152243A, methoxymorpholinyl DX) is a derivative of DX, 70-times more potent than DX that, although structurally similar, differs substantially for the mechanism of action, the pattern of resistance and metabolism. Unlike DX, nemorubicin is not sensitive to the expression of membrane glycoproteins important for the efflux of the drug and then exceeds the MDR1 resistance often observable with DX derivatives. Based on drug metabolism studies and the high therapeutic response rate observed in HCC patients receiving IHA administration of the drug during clinical trials, nemorubicin may be considered a good choice for locoregional treatment of HCC.

DCBeads™ are spherical microparticles, formulated into beads of varying size, which the presence of anionic charges enables them to interact with positively charged drugs, such as DX. Microspheres can both target their drug cargo by physical trapping in blood vessels and sustain the action of a therapeutic agent through controlled in situ release and clinical studies have showed that TACE with DCBeads™ loaded with DX is an effective and safe procedure in the treatment of HCC patients

The present study was undertaken to obtain preclinical data on the possible use of nemorubicin-loaded DCBeads™ for tumor chemotherapy and embolization. The main objectives of this study were the evaluation of the kinetics of loading and release of nemorubicin into and from DCBeads™, the assessment of the size and spherical shape of DCBeads™ upon nemorubicin loading, and the cytotoxic activity of the released nemorubicin towards tumor cells, in comparison with DX.

Nemorubicin loading into DCBeads™ was fast with a loading rate similar to DX. Conversely, DX showed a slower kinetic and a relevant amount of unreleased (97%) compound. The released drugs maintained the same antiproliferative activities on tumor cells that the unloaded drugs. Morphometric analysis of DCBeads™ during loading and release studies showed that, unlike DX, nemorubicin did not alter the physical characteristics of microspheres that maintain their shape and volume thus preserving their foreseen embolic potential. DCBeads™ are easily loaded with nemorubicin at clinically applicable dosages; loading and elution data support considering nemorubicin a suitable drug for TACE through microspheres.

Chapter 3 – Doxorubicin (DOX), an anticancer anthracycline antibiotic, is widely used in varieties of neoplastic diseases, such as leukemia, lymphomas, and solid tumors of the lung and breast. The most well known toxicity of anthracycline is its cardiac and cardiovascular toxicity. Without exception, clinical use of doxorubicin is limited by its cumulative and dose-dependent cardiomyopathy and congestive heart failure. The acute side effects of DOX treatment, such as myelosuppression, nausea, vomiting, pericarditis, myocarditis, and arrhythmia, are generally reversible and clinically manageable. As congestive heart failure is irreversible and life-threaten to patients with chronic DOX treatment, the prognosis and management of the congestive heart failure becomes critical. Several mechanisms such as free radical-dependent lipid peroxidation, mitochondrial dysfunction, calcium overload, and inhibition of membrane bound molecules have been reported for the DOX cardiotoxicity. This chapter provides an update to the pathological mechanism of DOX-induced cardiotoxicity. We also review and compare strategies in the management of DOX cardiotoxicity.

Chapter 4 – Doxorubicin (DOX) is classical but useful antitumor agent. DOX is used for the treatment of a variety of malignancies including solid tumors and leukemia due to its broad spectrum antitumor activity. However, DOX-induced cardiac toxicity as its adverse reaction is a dose limiting factor. Namely, DOX has double-edged effect with utilized action and severe adverse reaction. To make the most of ability of DOX, it is necessary to advance its therapy.

One of the advanced therapies is treatment of liposomal DOX. Liposomes are the principal means of effectively using medicines and are broadly recognized as a drug delivery system (DDS) carrier. However, liposomes after intravenous injection are rapidly taken up by reticuloendothelial system (RES) cells in the liver and spleen. This phenomenon reduces the effectiveness of liposomes as a drug carrier. Therefore, techniques for avoiding catch by RES cells and increasing the effectivity of liposomes based on polyethyleneglycol (PEG) modification on the surface of liposomes have been developed. DOX entrapped liposome by PEG modification induced an increase in the DOX level in the plasma and tumor and a decrease in this level in the liver. In vitro, The high entrapped amount of DOX into liposome demonstrated the usefulness of DOX liposomes for tumor cell uptake. Furthermore, anchor length of PEG-lipid on liposomal surface was clarified to be important on liposomal DOX uptake into tumor cell. The therapeutic index on peritoneal dissemination was influenced by particle size of liposomal DOX. The efficacy of liposomal DOX by modification using a mixture of PEG2000 and PEG with short PEG-chain was superior.

Another advanced therapy is biochemical modulation by foods or their components, not combined medicines. Theanine (specific amino acid in green tea) significantly enhanced the inhibitory effect of DOX on tumor growth and increased the DOX concentration in the tumor, and then the oral administration of theanine or green tea similarly enhanced the antitumor activity of DOX. Moreover, the combined theanine with DOX suppressed the hepatic metastasis of ovarian sarcoma. It was revealed that these effects by theanine were novel mechanism of enhancement of antitumor efficacy of DOX via the inhibition of glutamate transporters.

Anserine (a dipeptide contained in fowl and migratory fish) was increased DOX induced antitumor activity with the elevation of DOX concentration in the tumor. Anserine considered to take into tumor cells via a dipeptide transporter, and it resulted in an increase of the DOX influx in tumor cells.

Taurine (a major amino acid in fish and meat) and cucurbitacin E and I (a bitter tasting component of squash fruit) co-treatment was confirmed to increase DOX induced antitumor activity without an increase in adverse reactions by DOX, too. Namely, it was clarified that some foods and their components were useful as a modulator to enhance the therapeutic index of cancer patients and improve quality of life.

In conclusion, advanced therapies of DOX by liposomalization of DOX or combined food components with DOX was expected to contribute to cancer chemotherapy.

Chapter 5 – Despite the constant development of new drugs and biologic agents that have been introduced into cancer therapeutics, for decades doxorubicin (Doxo) remains the frontline drug against cancers, sarcomas, and hematological malignancies. Unfortunately, doxorubicin is not specifically targeting tumor agent and it also affects healthy tissues.

According to World Health Organization, breast cancer (BC) is the most frequent solid tumor in women worldwide, affecting more than a million subjects every year. Although it is well recognized that there are several molecular BC subtypes responsive to specific antineoplastic therapy, which is the step forward to individualized treatment, chemotherapy, including Doxo, is still indicated in the majority of BC patients. BC is a curable disease if it is diagnosed in early stages and afterwards treated with adjuvant full dose-intensity Doxo chemotherapy. This gives special importance to the strategy for prevention and management of its side effects. Successful use of Doxo is interrupted with a wide spectrum of toxicities, including acute nausea and vomiting, cardiotoxicity, myelosuppression, hepatotoxicity, gastrointestinal problems, renal toxicity and brain toxicity as usually seen in clinical practice. The main reason for Doxo withdrawal in BC patients is chemotherapy–induced emesis, while the major concern in the decision making process about continuation of treatment is Doxo–induced cardiotoxicity. Doxo is never applied as a single drug to BC patients, but most frequently in combination with cyclophosphamide (AC regimen). The AC regimen is recently recognized as highly-emetogenic, especially in younger women, despite the fact that each drug in this combination is of moderate emetogenic potential. Because of that the proper antiemetic prophylaxis is mandatory, including the use of NK1 and 5HT3 inhibitors, besides corticosteroids. Because heart damage is the greatest risk of Doxo-induced toxicity its administration must be dose-limited. If a lifetime accumulation of Doxo exceeds the recommended 450 mg/m^2, 50% of patients would experience measurable functional impairment, while more than 26% of them would develop congestive heart failure. Several approaches have been tested with the attempt to lower the risk of cardiac damage, such as Doxo administration as 96h infusion, liposomal Doxo delivery system, and various cardioprotective agents.

In this review we will summarize evidence and facts on prevention and management of Doxo cardiotoxicity, nausea and vomiting, based on literature data and our experience.

In: Doxorubicin
Editor: Melinda Pache
ISBN: 978-1-63117-233-5

Chapter 1

INTRAPERITONEAL DOXORUBICIN: RATIONALE, PHARMACOKINETIC STUDIES AND CLINICAL RESULTS

Paul H. Sugarbaker[*]
Washington Cancer Institute, MedStar Washington Hospital Center, Washington, DC, US

ABSTRACT

Background: Doxorubicin is a cancer chemotherapy agent with a wide spectrum of activity to a variety of cancers. It also has well known toxic side effects that must be minimized for its successful use clinically. A narrow therapeutic window exists for optimal cancer effects combined with an acceptable toxicity.

Materials and Methods: The application of doxorubicin in the prevention and treatment of peritoneal metastases from colorectal, gastric, and ovarian cancer plus peritoneal mesothelioma has been extensively published. Morbidity and mortality assessments have been recorded. High pressure liquid chromatography has been used to determine drug distribution into peritoneal fluid, plasma, normal and cancerous tissues and urine following doxorubicin administration into the peritoneal space.

[*] Corresponding author: Paul H. Sugarbaker, MD, FACS, FRCS, Washington Cancer Institute, 106 Irving St., NW, Suite 3900, Washington, DC 20010 USA, Tel: 202-877-3908, Fax: 202-877-8602, Email: Paul.Sugarbaker@medstar.net.

A large volume of chemotherapy solution has been used to widely distribute the drug to peritoneal surfaces.
Results: Intraperitoneal doxorubicin has been studied in a rat model to determine pharmacokinetic parameters in mammals, possible augmentation by hyperthermia and by pressure. Clinical data in patients has established the parameters for safe drug delivery. Pharmacokinetic studies in humans confirm the favorable pharmacology of intraperitoneal drug delivery for peritoneal metastases patients. The treatment of a large number of patients by early postoperative intraperitoneal drug delivery or by hyperthermic intraoperative drug delivery establishes the clinical utility of this route of administration. Clinical studies in patients with sarcoma, appendiceal malignancy, and colorectal cancer have established this drug in combination with other chemotherapy agents as a standard of care.

Conclusions: Doxorubicin shows characteristics favorable for intracavitary administration and toxicity studies suggest that it is well tolerated by the intraperitoneal route after a major surgical procedure. On the basis of pharmacologic and clinical studies, intraperitoneal doxorubicin has become a global standard of care for hyperthermic perioperative chemotherapy for the management of mesothelioma, sarcoma, appendiceal malignancy, and colorectal cancer with peritoneal metastases.

INTRODUCTION

In the past, all adjuvant and neoadjuvant chemotherapy treatments were administered via the intravenous route. Not only the systemic but also the local-regional destruction of cancerous tissue was assumed to be optimal by this route of administration. Also, the systemic toxicities were considered unavoidable in order to achieve the desired cytotoxic effects. As clinical information regarding the anatomic sites of surgical treatment failure have accumulated, it has become clear that gastrointestinal and gynecologic malignancies have a continuing high incidence of local-regional and peritoneal surface progression. Indeed, the high rates of local-regional and peritoneal surface progression of pancreas cancer, gastric cancer, visceral and retroperitoneal sarcoma, and ovarian cancer may lead one to conclude that the current surgical approach to these diseases should be considered a failure. With the exception of ovarian cancer, the incidence of local-regional and peritoneal surface progression has not been improved by the use of systemic chemotherapy either prior to or after cancer resection.

In order to reduce the treatment failures within the field of surgical dissection and within the peritoneal cavity, suggestions regarding a new chemotherapy strategy have developed. This new approach is not neoadjuvant chemotherapy prior to surgery or after adjuvant chemotherapy to be used after surgery, but rather perioperative chemotherapy to be used as a planned part of the surgical intervention [1-4].

RATIONALE FOR PERIOPERATIVE CHEMOTHERAPY ADMINISTRATION

Gastrointestinal and gynecologic malignancies are diseases that spread through lymphatic channels, portal blood, and peritoneal spaces by single cells or microscopic multicellular nodules. As shown in Table 1, peritoneal metastases are present in 5-25% of patients prior to the primary cancer resection [5-8].

Table 1. Survey of the incidence of peritoneal metastases observed at the time of primary gastrointestinal cancer diagnosis

Primary Site	% Peritoneal Metastases	Reference
Colon	8.5	Sjo, JSO, 2011 (5)
Rectum	25.8	Shepard, J Clin Pathol, 1995 (6)
Stomach	5 - 20	Ikeguchi, Antica Res, 1994 (7)
Pancreas	26	Dragovich, Medscape, 2013 (8)

Attempts to Reduce the Incidence of Lymphatic Metastases Diagnosed in Follow-Up

The treatment strategy that will reliably interrupt subsequent progression of cancer implants within lymphatic channels and lymph nodes is a wide surgical removal of the relevant lymphatic system immediately adjacent to the primary cancer. This direct approach to lymphatic spread becomes increasingly effective the more extensive the lymphatic clearance that is performed [9, 10]. This has been shown to be true for colorectal and gastric cancer but does not seem to apply to pancreas malignancy [11]. It has been shown to prolong disease-free survival but not overall survival in ovarian cancer [12]. Further clinical trials with extensive lymphadenectomy in ovarian cancer are currently in progress [13]. It is possible that neoadjuvant systemic chemotherapy or chemoradiation therapy may reduce the extent of lymphatic dissemination prior to surgery and improve the clearance and containment provided by primary cancer resection. This preoperative treatment may be most important for low rectal cancer and gastric cancer [14, 15].

Attempts to Reduce the Incidence of Hepatic Metastases Diagnosed in Follow-Up

Attempts to reduce the progression of metastases in the liver for colorectal cancer were reported by Metzger and colleagues [16]. Their strategy was the direct infusion of 5-fluorouracil and mitomycin C chemotherapy into the liver through the portal vein. Their positive result may have been caused by the local-regional effects of chemotherapy within the liver or by systemic effects of these drugs. It is possible that neoadjuvant systemic chemotherapy can downsize and partially devitalize the primary cancer to reduce the likelihood of cancer emboli into the portal vein as a result of the trauma of surgery. This concept is an extension of the "no touch technique" originally advocated by Turnbull [17]. It is safe to conclude that, at this point in time, no strategy to prevent the recurrence of liver metastases diagnosed in follow-up exists.

Attempts to Reduce the Incidence of Peritoneal Metastases and Local-Regional Recurrence Diagnosed in Follow-Up

In contrast to liver metastases the surgeon's efforts during the operative event to eradicate subsequent peritoneal metastases and local-regional progression are more successful. The strategy combines innovative chemotherapy treatments with the primary surgical intervention. The rationale for the perioperative timing of intraperitoneal cancer chemotherapy administration is based on the tumor cell entrapment hypothesis (Figure 1). It provides an explanation for the low incidence of local-regional and peritoneal surface cancer nodules at the time of an R-0 cancer resection as compared to the high incidence of local-regional recurrence and peritoneal metastases observed during follow-up and at the time of diagnosis of recurrent disease [18-20]. There are two plausible explanations for this observation. First, microscopic cancer not appreciated by the surgeon at the time of resection frequently exists. Second, microscopic disease transmitted into the free peritoneal space or into the dissection site of the primary malignancy as a result of the trauma of the cancer resection may often occur. Although lymph node progression and hepatic metastases progression are more likely to be effectively treated by neoadjuvant or adjuvant systemic chemotherapy, peritoneal metastases and local-regional progression may be most effectively prevented by perioperative intraperitoneal and systemic chemotherapy.

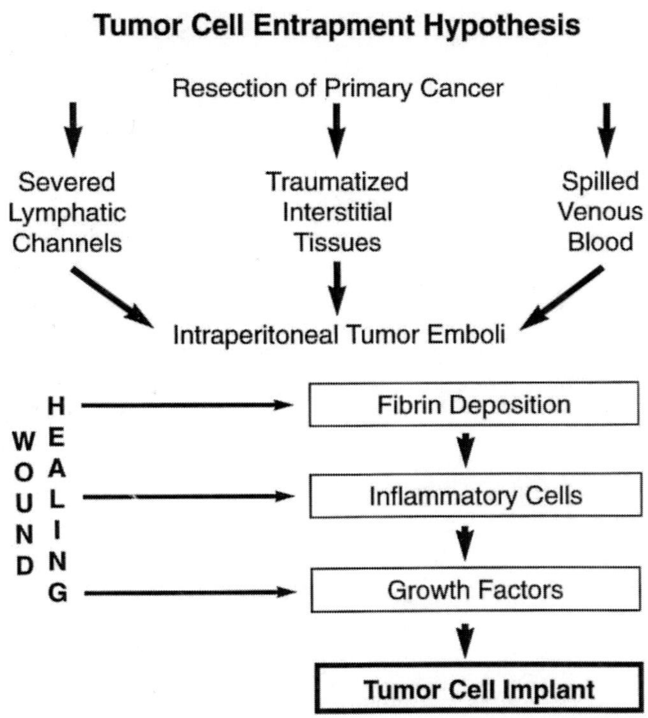

Figure 1. Tumor cell entrapment hypothesis.

Although current use of perioperative chemotherapy with primary gastrointestinal cancer is limited, recent reports are encouraging [21-24]. Normal epithelial cells exfoliate from the bowel surface as part of their normal life cycle. Cancer cells from gastrointestinal and ovarian primary malignancy may retain this capability when cancer cells are released from severed lymph channels, from traumatized primary cancer mass, or from severed portal blood vessels. These cancer cells have a high efficiency of implantation [25]. The malignant cells will implant at high density in and around the resection site as local recurrence and at lower density on distant peritoneal surfaces as peritoneal metastases. The incidence of surgical treatment failure as documented when surgery alone is used to treat the primary gastrointestinal malignancy is shown in Table 2.

Before cancer cells have the opportunity to implant and grow, perioperative chemotherapy may be used to destroy them. Access to all surfaces contaminated by exfoliated cancer cells will be facilitated by several unique possibilities offered by perioperative chemotherapy administration. First, an intraperitoneal route of administration in a large volume of carrier solution (usually 3 or 4 liters) is possible. This large volume of chemotherapy solution may come into direct contact with all abdominal and pelvic surfaces. Second, manual distribution of the large volume of intraperitoneal chemotherapy solution can guarantee repeated access of the cytotoxic solution to all abdominal and pelvic surfaces for an extended time period. It is possible to manipulate the intestines and abdominal and pelvic structures so that they are repeatedly in contact with the chemotherapy solution. Third, the timing of the chemotherapy administration is such that entrapment of the cancer cells in scar is avoided. In other words, the tumor cell entrapment as diagramed in Figure 1 should be prevented. To avoid tumor cell entrapment the intraperitoneal chemotherapy must be a planned part of the operative procedure in the early postoperative period (postoperative days 1-5) [1] or within the operating room as hyperthermic perioperative chemotherapy [26]. Fourth, moderate heat can be used to augment the cytotoxicity of the chemotherapy. Fifth and finally, systemic perioperative chemotherapy can be used to augment the complete clearance of cancer cells from peritoneal surfaces and the primary cancer resection site [27].

Doxorubicin is a chemotherapy agent that is non-cell cycle-specific, has a broad range of activity to gastrointestinal and gynecologic malignancy, and is compatible with combined administration of numerous other chemotherapy agents. It is definitely an agent that should be selected for study by perioperative administration into the peritoneal space. The purpose of this manuscript is to examine laboratory and clinical data regarding the uses of intraperitoneal doxorubicin to date, to review the global utilization of intraperitoneal doxorubicin for prevention and treatment of peritoneal metastases, and then propose possible future studies for its perioperative intraperitoneal utilization.

Table 2. Incidence of peritoneal metastases and local-regional progression observed in follow-up at the time of gastrointestinal cancer recurrence

Primary Site	% Peritoneal Metastases (Isolated)	% Peritoneal Metastases (Combined)	Reference
Colorectum	67	33	Jayne, BJS, 2002 (18)
Stomach	29	54	D'Angelica, MSKCC, 2004 (19)
Pancreas	15	61	Donohue, JHMI, 2009 (20)

LABORATORY DATA CONCERNING INTRAPERITONEAL DOXORUBICIN

Pharmacokinetic studies of doxorubicin in a murine ovarian cancer model were reported by Ozols and colleagues [28]. They compared drug delivery by intraperitoneal and intravenous administration. Doxorubicin-specific intranuclear fluorescence was detected in ascites tumor cells within 1 minute following an intraperitoneal dose but was undetectable at any time following an equitoxic intravenous dose. Doxorubicin-specific fluorescence was observed after an intraperitoneal dose in all the tumor cells coating the diaphragm. After an intravenous dose, there was only faint and patchy intranuclear fluorescence in tumor cells coating the diaphragm.

The visual observations were confirmed by measurement of tissue doxorubicin levels. Over a 48-hour period, the concentration of doxorubicin and its fluorescent metabolites after intraperitoneal administration exceeded by at least 1 log the intravenous drug level in ascites fluid, with a peak intraperitoneal level (7.5 μg/ml) almost 30 times higher than the peak intravenous level (0.26 μg/ml). In the tumor cells, the peak level was 50 times higher after an intraperitoneal dose, and at least a 1-log differential between intravenous and intraperitoneal levels was maintained throughout the 48 hours studied. In contrast, the peak drug levels in heart, liver, and kidney were markedly higher after the intravenous route than after the intraperitoneal route, with ratios of 3:1 for heart and kidney and 8:1 for liver. The differential in tissue concentrations rapidly decreased, so that by 24 hours there was no difference in drug concentration between the routes in any of the three organs.

Pharmacokinetic studies of intraperitoneal doxorubicin in an animal model were continued by Jacquet and colleagues [29]. They studied a 2 mg/kg intraperitoneal infusion of 300 ml dialysis solution over 60 minutes in a rat model. The peak peritoneal fluid level was 2.98±0.16 μg /ml and the peak plasma level was 0.04±0.01 μg /ml. The intraperitoneal levels of doxorubicin achieved and even surpassed those levels required for destruction of cancer cells from large number of malignancies [30]. Their studies documented the marked increase in local-regional exposure of the doxorubicin. Over the 90 minutes, the area under the curve ratio (AUC ratio) of peritoneal fluid AUC to plasma AUC was 87.9±37.8. This study documented that the clearance (metabolism) of doxorubicin from the plasma was more rapid than escape of doxorubicin from the peritoneal space over the 60 minutes of the experiment. These data suggested that doxorubicin may be an ideal cancer chemotherapy agent that would combine intense intraperitoneal cytotoxic effects with a low level of systemic toxicity [31].

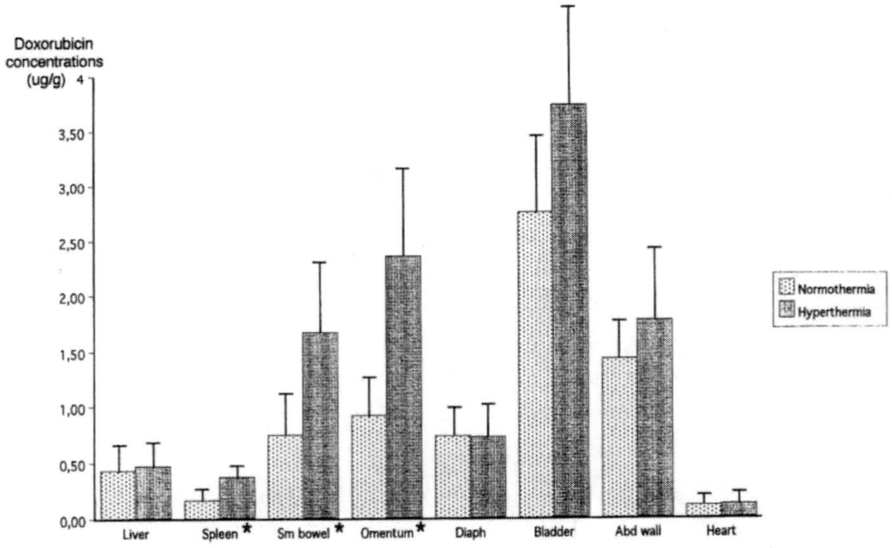

Figure 2. Doxorubicin concentrations in tissues after 1 hour of normothermic (⊡) or hyperthermic (■) intraperitoneal infusion. (From reference 29 with permission).

Hyperthermia did increase the concentration of aglycones in plasma, liver, and bladder. This may be related to increased portal blood flow through the liver under hyperthermic conditions [32].

Jacquet and colleagues went on to study the effects of hyperthermia on intraperitoneal doxorubicin administration [29]. The pharmacokinetic effects of hyperthermia on aglycones was also determined. The peak peritoneal fluid levels, peak plasma levels, peritoneal fluid AUC, plasma AUC, and AUC ratios did not differ for chemotherapy solution at 36.4°C (±0.6) as compared to chemotherapy solution at 42.5°C (±0.8). Aglycones were not detectable in peritoneal fluid; however, with hyperthermia the concentration of aglycones was significantly higher in plasma ($p<0.001$) and plasma AUC ($p<0.001$).

After the 1-hour peritoneal lavage with doxorubicin, multiple tissues were harvested from normothermic and hyperthermic treated rats. Figure 2 shows that tissues contained within the peritoneal space and bathed on all sides by chemotherapy solution (spleen, small bowel, and omentum) had significantly higher doxorubicin concentrations with hyperthermia while systemic organs (liver, diaphragm, bladder, abdominal wall, and heart) had similar concentrations with and without intraperitoneal heat.

Doxorubicin Penetration into Normal and Cancerous Tissues

Los and McVie summarized the data available up to 1990 concerning chemotherapy delivery by intraperitoneal administration [33]. Studies with doxorubicin as a single and as a multi-agent treatment were reviewed. They emphasized the high incidence of resection site and peritoneal surface disease observed in patients in whom cancer recurred. In their report, experimental data regarding tumor penetration by cytostatic drugs was carefully reviewed. Intraperitoneal drug delivery to cancerous tissue was dependent on drug penetration by diffusion due to concentration differences (concentration gradient), duration of exposure, and removal of drug by capillary blood flow. Based on these observations, any advantage intraperitoneal chemotherapy will have over intravenous administration will be limited to those clinical situations in which small-volume disease is present at the start of treatment.

Ozols and colleagues studied intraperitoneal doxorubicin in a murine model [28]. Doxorubicin intraperitoneally penetrated only into the outermost 4 to 6 layers of intraabdominal tumors, whereas the intravenous route doxorubicin-specific fluorescence was observed in a patchy distribution throughout the tumor.

Attempts to Increase Doxorubicin Penetration into Tissues Using Pressure

In the model of intraperitoneal drug delivery presented by Dedrick and colleagues, cancer chemotherapy entered normal and cancerous tissues by simple diffusion [31]. Drugs enter normal or cancerous tissues as a result of the large concentration difference within the peritoneal space as compared to the plasma compartment. In an attempt to increase doxorubicin penetration into tissue, Jacquet and colleagues studied the effects of increased intraabdominal pressure [34]. These data were obtained in a rat model. Increased intraabdominal pressure of 10, 20, and 30 mg Hg did not change the pharmacokinetics of intraperitoneal doxorubicin. Also, high intraabdominal pressures of 20 or 30 mg Hg were associated with visible intestinal ischemia after the 60 minutes of treatment. Doxorubicin concentrations in tissues at 30 mm Hg showed increased drug levels in parietal peritoneal tissues from abdominal wall, bladder, and diaphragm at 10 minutes but this increase was not sustained at 60 minutes. The data failed to show increased doxorubicin uptake in tissues covered by visceral peritoneum (spleen, small bowel, and omentum). These authors concluded that increased intraabdominal pressure had a transient effect on doxorubicin penetration into parietal peritoneal tissues and none into visceral peritoneal tissues.

Studies to Determine the Safety of Intraperitoneal Doxorubicin

The sclerotic effects of doxorubicin are well known and the dangers of drug infiltration into tissues surrounding intravenous infusion sites are well described [35]. Litterst and colleagues simulated the "belly bath" treatments in a rat model [36]. Fifty milliliters of various concentrations of drug solution was administered intraperitoneally and was allowed to remain in situ for either 4 or 36 hours prior to removal. Animals were analyzed at 2, 14, and 60 days after treatment. A wide dose range from lethal to nontoxic was used. The most common lesion in surviving animals was chronic fibrosing peritonitis. Peritoneal adhesions were the most commonly observed finding when higher concentrations (20-150 μg/ml) were used for 4 hours. Commonly observed systemic toxic effects (bone marrow, gastrointestinal tract, and heart) were not seen in this study.

Sugarbaker performed dose escalation studies with intraperitoneal doxorubicin as early postoperative intraperitoneal chemotherapy (EPIC) for the first five days after a resection of abdominal or pelvic neoplasm [37, 38]. Also, a single cycle of delayed intraperitoneal doxorubicin was pharmacologically studied. The dose escalations were accompanied by second-look surgery in order to determine the extent of peritoneal sclerosis caused by the sclerotic effects of doxorubicin in patients who had undergone major cancer surgery. These authors determined that 0.1 mg/kg in 1 to 1.5 liters of a 1.5% dextrose peritoneal dialysis solution given for 5 consecutive days postoperatively was well tolerated. A thin layer of fibrosis was evident at the time of second-look surgery but bowel function continued as normal. A single patient given two cycles of intraperitoneal chemotherapy developed peritoneal sclerosis requiring parenteral feeding to maintain adequate hydration and nutrition.

The total dose of intraperitoneal doxorubicin over 5 days was between 25 and 35 mg (0.1 mg/kg for 5 consecutive days). For hyperthermic intraperitoneal chemotherapy (HIPEC), the total dose determined as safe over the 90 minutes of treatment was 15 mg/m^2. The drug was used in 1.5% dextrose peritoneal dialysis solution with a volume of chemotherapy solution of 1.5 L/m^2. With HIPEC as well with EPIC, between 25 and 35 mg total dose of doxorubicin is recommended with this dose range being adjusted for the patient's total body surface area.

As HIPEC treatment has been modified over two decades, multi-agent chemotherapy utilizing doxorubicin has been used in the Peritoneal Surface Oncology Program at the Medstar Washington Cancer Institute. HIPEC with mitomycin C at 15 mg/m^2 and doxorubicin at 15 mg/m^2 has been used with an open technique for a 90-minute hyperthermic peritoneal lavage at 41.5 to 42.5°C [39]. Although reoperation for postoperative adhesions was required in 5% of 560 patients, only a single instance of severe peritoneal sclerosis has been recorded. Reoperative surgery was performed in this single patient with complete success with restoration of normal oral nutrition and hydration.

Also, HIPEC with cisplatin at 50 mg/m^2 and doxorubicin at 15 mg/m^2 has been used with an open technique for a 90-minute hyperthermic peritoneal lavage at 41.5 to 42.5°C [39]. Reoperation for adhesion was required in 5% of 380 patients. A single patient at the time of reoperation was observed to have extensive peritoneal fibrosis thought to be related to intraperitoneal chemotherapy administration. Reoperative surgery in this patient was extensive and required an ostomy because of dense fibrosis surrounding small bowel. However, ostomy closure after 6 months was successful and the patient has been restored to normal oral nutrition and hydration.

Ozols and colleague performed phase I and pharmacologic studies with repeated instillations of doxorubicin in patients with progressive ovarian malignancy [40]. Two liters of intraperitoneal drug was used with concentrations of 9-54 μmol. Their maximal dose of 50 μmol was 60 mg in 2 liters of 1.5% dextrose peritoneal dialysis solution. As a result of toxicity studies, they recommended repeated instillations at 2-week intervals of 30-40 mg of doxorubicin in 2 liters of dialysis solution. In short term follow-up, Ozols and colleagues report no instances of drug-induced intestinal obstruction although 2 patients had an increase in asymptomatic abdominal adhesions noted at a second-look laparotomy and at a restaging peritonoscopy. However, long-term follow-up of the 10 patients in their study regarding intestinal function is not available. Abdominal pain was the major dose limiting toxicity during the study period. Some of the patients who survived their ovarian cancer as a result of the intraperitoneal doxorubicin did require long-term parenteral nutrition and reoperative surgical procedures in an attempt to relieve "a frozen abdomen" from progressive scar tissue. The incidence of profound peritoneal sclerosis in this group of patients with long-term follow-up is not available.

Rossi and coworkers studied hyperthermic intraperitoneal intraoperative chemotherapy combined with cytoreductive surgery [41]. They conducted a phase I study with doxorubicin and cisplatin in patients with peritoneal carcinomatosis or sarcomatosis in 31 patients. Maximum tolerated dose was 15.25 mg/L for doxorubicin. The perfusate/plasma area under the curve ratio was favorable at 162±113. There were no postoperative deaths. Surgery-related complications were observed in 25% of cases.

A summary of the toxicity studies of intraperitoneal doxorubicin suggest that a maximum dose for a single instillation is 15 mg/m^2. Repeated instillations of intraperitoneal doxorubicin are not recommended. Doxorubicin can be combined with other cancer chemotherapy agents such as mitomycin C and cisplatin with a high degree of safety and an expected increased efficacy. Moderate heat (41.5 - 42.5°C) does not increase the sclerotic effects of intraperitoneal doxorubicin.

PHARMACOKINETICS OF INTRAPERITONEAL DOXORUBICIN IN PATIENTS

Ozols and coworkers reported a maximal pharmacologic advantage (peak peritoneal concentration/peak plasma concentration) of 474 after an intraperitoneal dose of 40 mg in 2 liters of fluid [40]. The 4-hour peritoneal level was 166 times higher than the corresponding plasma level. The marked pharmacokinetic advantage of intraperitoneal administration observed in animal studies was confirmed in humans.

Sugarbaker and coworkers used doxorubicin under different clinical circumstances from Ozols et al; they worked with patients who had progressive ovarian cancer. Sugarbaker instilled the drug on postoperative days 1-5 after a major cytoreductive surgical procedure in patients who had gastrointestinal cancer or abdominal sarcoma. The surgery was designed to remove all visible evidence of peritoneal metastases. The drug was to treat residual disease not visible to the surgeon's naked eye. Because the drug was used for 5 consecutive days, lower doses at 0.1 mg/kg in two liters of fluid were used on a daily basis. The AUC ratio of peritoneal fluid to plasma was 230. In some patients, it was possible to obtain intraportal blood samples. The AUC ratio of portal to systemic drug was estimated at 5 (Figure 3). These studies documented the theoretical benefits of intraperitoneal doxorubicin administration for cancer on peritoneal surfaces but also suggested some benefit for treatment of metastatic disease within the liver [37].

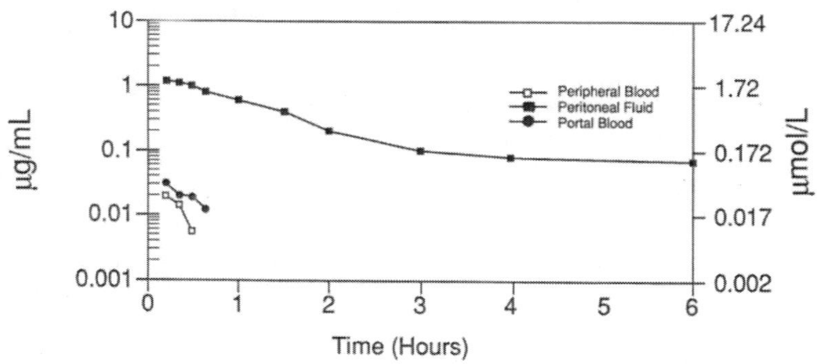

Figure 3. Doxorubicin pharmacokinetic study after intraperitoneal administration one day after major cytoreductive surgery. The dose was 2.5 mg in 2 liters of 1.5% dextrose peritoneal dialysis solution. The treatment was continued for five days. (From reference 37 with permission)

IMPACT OF SURGICAL AND CLINICAL FACTORS ON THE PHARMACOLOGY OF HYPERTHERMIC INTRAPERITONEAL DOXORUBICIN ADMINISTRATION

Sugarbaker and colleagues studied the pharmacology of 145 consecutive colorectal or appendiceal metastases patients who were treated with cytoreductive surgery prior to treatment with HIPEC with doxorubicin as a part of a multi-drug regimen [42]. A single bolus administration of doxorubicin at 15 mg/m^2 in 1.5% dextrose peritoneal dialysis solution was used. With HIPEC the AUC ratio of peritoneal fluid to plasma was 78. At 90 minutes, 12% of the drug remained in the chemotherapy solution and 88% was retained by the body. Extensive peritonectomy increased the rate of clearance of doxorubicin from the peritoneal space by approximately 15%. Extensive visceral resection such as total colectomy or total gastrectomy decreased the clearance of doxorubicin from the peritoneal space by decreasing the total diffusion surface. Also, a decreased clearance of doxorubicin from the peritoneal space was noted in those patients who had a contracted abdomen as a result of extensive prior surgery. If the total volume of chemotherapy within the peritoneal space was reduced, the total diffusion surface was reduced and this resulted in a reduced clearance of doxorubicin from the peritoneal space.

Van der Speeten and colleagues showed that doxorubicin placed into the peritoneal space under hyperthermic conditions developed higher levels within peritoneal tumor nodules or normal peritoneal tissues than in the peritoneal fluid [43]. This suggested a non-reversible binding of doxorubicin within tissue. An increased amount of fibrous tissue within a cancer nodule reduced this enhanced uptake of chemotherapy. The highest uptake was noted within mucinous malignancies. When hyperthermic intraperitoneal doxorubicin was compared to hyperthermic intrapleural administration of doxorubicin, a markedly reduced clearance of drug from the pleural space was noted. These authors hypothesize that the visceral peritoneum within the abdomen was the major site for doxorubicin clearance. Parietal peritoneum or parietal pleura had less blood supply than the visceral peritoneum and therefore cleared doxorubicin more slowly.

Clinical Use of Doxorubicin with Debilitating Cancerous Ascites

Ozols and colleagues reported that intraperitoneal doxorubicin caused a marked reduction in ascites production in ovarian cancer patients. Patients having 3-5 liters of ascites production per week and requiring frequent paracentesis had no further need for therapeutic paracentesis after a single cycle of intraperitoneal doxorubicin. The cytotoxic effects of the drug combined with its sclerotic effects most likely combined to produce this remarkable resolution of malignant ascites by this drug [40].

Current Global Utilization of Intraperitoneal Doxorubicin

Currently, doxorubicin is a part of multi-agent hyperthermic intraperitoneal chemotherapy at many institutions around the world. It is most commonly used along with mitomycin C or with cisplatin [39]. Toxicities are minimal and at the dose of 15 mg/m^2 it is well tolerated with peritoneal sclerosis seen as an extremely unusual event. The concentration of the chemotherapy solution in the patient who is 2 m^2 would be 10 mg/L. The peritoneal surface oncology program at the Istituto Tumori in Milan, Italy uses a very similar concentration of doxorubicin along with cisplatin. The diseases treated include gastric cancer, colorectal cancer, peritoneal mesothelioma, and ovarian malignancy. In patients treated at Medstar Washington Cancer Institute, the cisplatin and doxorubicin are given intraperitoneal along with ifosfamide as a systemic chemotherapy agent designed for heat targeting to peritoneal surfaces [39]. Despite being an “old chemotherapy agent”, its efficacy remains important and with proper dosimetry its safety as an intraperitoneal drug has been repeatedly demonstrated. Currently, as a part of a multi-agent intraperitoneal chemotherapy regimen, doxorubicin has global application.

Future Studies for Perioperative Utilization of Intraperitoneal Doxorubicin

The major challenge that remains for the clinician researcher regards the optimal methodology for intraperitoneal doxorubicin administration. Should it be as a hyperthermic treatment as a planned part of the surgical procedure known as HIPEC or should it be used in the early postoperative period in a treatment known as EPIC? No direct comparisons of HIPEC doxorubicin with EPIC doxorubicin are available.

In administering doxorubicin with HIPEC, the open technique which allows for manual distribution of the drug has not been compared with the closed technique that relies on abdominal distention for drug distribution. In a comparison of the open and closed techniques, Sugarbaker suggested that the adverse events were less using manual manipulation and that there were less anastomotic leaks. More uniform drug distribution may account for this increased safety [44].

Finally, the proper drug combinations utilizing multiple intraperitoneal chemotherapy agents combined with systemic chemotherapy need to be investigated. The cancer nodule can be accessed by simple diffusion through intraperitoneal chemotherapy administration and also directly by intravenous administration. Most likely, the optimal combinations will be bidirectional, that is, with both via intravenous and intraperitoneal delivery of drugs best pharmacologically suited for one route of administration over the other [27].

References

[1] Sugarbaker, PH; Graves, T; DeBruijn, EA; et al. Early postoperative intraperitoneal chemotherapy as an adjuvant therapy to surgery for peritoneal carcinomatosis from gastrointestinal cancer: Pharmacologic studies. *Cancer Res*, 1990, 50, 5790-5794.

[2] Sugarbaker, PH. Successful management of microscopic residual disease in large bowel cancer. *Cancer Chemother Pharmacol*, 1999, 43(Suppl), S15-S25.

[3] Sugarbaker, PH. Management of peritoneal surface malignancy: The surgeon's role. *Langenbeck's Arch Surg*, 1999, 384, 576-587.

[4] Sugarbaker, PH; (Ed). Cytoreductive Surgery & Perioperative Chemotherapy for Peritoneal Surface Malignancy. Textbook and Video Atlas. Cine-Med Publishing: *Woodbury*, CT, 2012.

[5] Sjo, OH; Berg, M; Merok, MA; et al. Peritoneal carcinomatosis of colon cancer origin: Highest incidence in women and in patients with right-sided tumors. *J Surg Oncol*, 2011, 104, 792-797.

[6] Shepherd, NA; Baxter, KJ; Love, SB. Influence of local peritoneal involvement on pelvic recurrence and prognosis in rectal cancer. *J Clin Pathol*, 1995, 48, 849-855.

[7] Ikeguchi, M; Oka, A; Tsujitani, S; Maeta, M; Kaibara, N. Relationship between area of serosal invasion and intraperitoneal free cancer cells in patients with gastric cancer. *Anticancer Res.*, 1994, 14(5B), 2131-2134.

[8] Dragovich, T. (2013, October 14) Pancreatic Cancer. *Medscape*. Retrieved 11/22/2013 from http://emedicine.medscape.com/article/280605-overview.

[9] Swanson, RS; Compton, CC; Stewart, AK; Bland, KI. The prognosis of T3N0 colon cancer is dependent on the number of lymph nodes examined. *Ann Surg Oncol*, 2003,10(1), 65-71.

[10] Le Voyer, TE; Sigurdson, ER; Hanlon, AL; et al. Colon cancer survival is associated with increasing number of lymph nodes analyzed: a secondary survey of intergroup trial INT-0089. *J Clin Oncol*, 2003, 21(15), 2912-2919.

[11] Pedrazzoli, S; DiCarlo, V; Dionigo, R; et al. Standard versus extended lymphadenectomy associated with pancreatoduodenectomy in the surgical treatment of adenocarcinoma of the head of the pancreas: a multicenter, prospective, randomized study. Lymphadenectomy Study Group. *Ann Surg*, 1998, 228(4), 508-517.

[12] Panici, PB; Maggioni, A; Hacker, N; et al. Systematic aortic and pelvic lymphadenectomy versus resection of bulky nodes only in optimally debulked advanced ovarian cancer: a randomized clinical trial. *J Natl Cancer Inst*, 2005, 20, 97(8), 560-566.

[13] Lymphadenectomy In Ovarian Neoplasms (LION). ClinicalTrials.gov Identifier: NCT00712218. http://www.clinicaltrials.gov/show/NCT00712218.

[14] Peeters, KC; Marijnen, CA; Nagtegaal, ID; et al. The TME trial after a median follow-up of 6 years: Increased local control but not survival benefit in irradiated patients with resectable rectal carcinoma. *Ann Surg*, 2007, 246, 693-701.

[15] Ychou, M; Boige, V; Pignon, JP; et al. Perioperative chemotherapy compared with surgery alone for resectable gastroesophageal adenocarcinoma: An FNCLCC and FFCD multicenter phase III trial. *J Clin Oncol*, 2011, 29, 1715-1721.

[16] Laffer, U; Metzger, U; Aeberhard, P; et al. Adjuvant perioperative portal vein or peripheral intravenous chemotherapy for potentially curative colorectal cancer: long-term results of a randomized controlled trial. *Int J Colorectal Dis*, 2008, 23, 1233-1241.

[17] Turnbull, RB; Kyle, K; Watson, FR; et al. Cancer of the colon: The influence of the no-touch isolation technic on survival rates. *Ann Surg*, 1967, 166, 420-427.

[18] Jayne, DG; Fook, S; Loi, C; Seow-Choen, F. Peritoneal carcinomatosis from colorectal cancer. *Br J Surg*, 2002, 89, 1545-1550.

[19] D'Angelica, M; Gonen, M; Brennan, MF; Turnbull, AD; Bains, M; Karpeh, MS. Patterns of initial recurrence in completely resected gastric adenocarcinoma. *Ann Surg*, 2004, 240(5), 808-816.

[20] Iacobuzio-Donahue, CA; Fu, B; Yachida, S; et al. DPC4 gene status of the primary carcinoma correlates with patterns of failure in patients with pancreatic cancer. *J Clin Oncol*, 2009, 27(11), 1806-1813.

[21] Pestieau, SR; Sugarbaker, PH. Treatment of primary colon cancer with peritoneal carcinomatosis: A comparison of concomitant versus delayed management. *Dis Colon Rectum*, 2000, 43, 1341-1348.

[22] Sammartino, P; Sibio, S; Accarpio, F; Di Giorgio, A. Long-term results after proactive management for locoregional control in patients with colonic cancer at high risk of peritoneal metastases. (submitted for publication)

[23] Braam, HJ; Boerma, D; Wiezer, MJ; van Ramshorst, B. Hyperthermic perioperative chemotherapy during primary tumour resection limits extent of bowel resection compared to two-stage treatment. *Eur J Surg Oncol*, 2013, 39(9), 988-993.

[24] Yan, TD; Black, D; Sugarbaker, PH; et al. A systematic review and meta-analysis of the randomized controlled trials on adjuvant intraperitoneal chemotherapy for resectable gastric cancer. *Ann Surg Oncol*, 2007,14(10), 2702-2713.

[25] Weiss, L; (Ed). Principles of Metastasis. Academic Press, Inc: Orlando, FL, 1985.

[26] Glehen, O; Gilly, FN; Boutitie, F; et al. Toward curative treatment of peritoneal carcinomatosis from nonovarian origin by cytoreductive surgery combined with perioperative intraperitoneal chemotherapy. A

multi-institutional study of 1290 patients. *Cancer*, 2010,116, 5608-5618.

[27] Van der Speeten, K; Stuart, OA; Sugarbaker, PH. Pharmacology of perioperative cancer chemotherapy. (In) Sugarbaker PH (Ed). Cytoreductive Surgery & Perioperative Chemotherapy for Peritoneal Surface Malignancy. Textbook and Video Atlas. Cine-Med Publishing: Woodbury, CT, 2012, 159-182.

[28] Ozols, R; Locker, GY; Doroshow, JH; et al. Pharmacokinetics of adriamycin and tissue penetration in murine ovarian cancer. *Cancer Res*, 1979, 39, 3209-3214.

[29] Jacquet, P; Averbach, A; Stuart, OA; Chang, D; Sugarbaker, PH. Hyperthermic intraperitoneal doxorubicin: Pharmacokinetics, metabolism, and tissue distribution in a rat model. *Cancer Chemother Pharmacol*, 1998, 41(2), 147-154.

[30] Park, JG; Kramer, BS; Steinberg, SM; et al. Chemosensitivity testing of human colorectal carcinoma cell lines using a tetrazolium-based colorimetric assay. *Cancer Res*, 1987, 47(22), 5875-5879.

[31] Dedrick, RL. Theoretical and experimental bases of intraperitoneal chemotherapy. *Semin Oncol*, 1985, 12(3 Suppl. 4), 1-6.

[32] Karran, S. Progress in the assessment of liver blood flow in health and disease. *J R Coll Surg Edinb*, 1990, 35, 207-217.

[33] Los, G; McVie, JG. Experimental and clinical status of intraperitoneal chemotherapy. *Eur J Cancer*, 1990, 26, 755-762.

[34] Jacquet, P; Stuart, OA; Chang, D; Sugarbaker, PH. Effects of intra-abdominal pressure on pharmacokinetics and tissue distribution of doxorubicin after intraperitoneal administration. *Anti-cancer Drugs*, 1996, 7, 596-603.

[35] Dorr, RT; Alberts, DS; Chen, G. Experimental model of doxorubicin extravasation in the mouse. *J Pharmacol Methods*, 1980, 4, 237-250.

[36] Litterst, CL; Collins, JM; Lowe, MC; Arnold, ST; Powell, DM; Guarino, AM. Local and systemic toxicity resulting from large-volume Ip administration of doxorubicin in the rat. *Cancer Treat Rep*, 1982, 66, 157-161.

[37] Sugarbaker, PH. Early postoperative intraperitoneal adriamycin as an adjuvant treatment for visceral and retroperitoneal sarcoma. (In) Sugarbaker PH (ed); Peritoneal Carcinomatosis: Drugs and Diseases. Kluwer: Boston, 1996, 7-14.

[38] Sugarbaker, PH; Sweatman, TW; Graves, T; Cunliffe, W; Israel, M. Early postoperative intraperitoneal adriamycin: Pharmacologic studies and a preliminary clinical report. *Reg Cancer Treat*, 1991, 4, 127-131.

[39] Sugarbaker, PH. An overview of peritonectomy, visceral resections, and perioperative chemotherapy for peritoneal surface malignancy. (In) Sugarbaker PH (Ed). Cytoreductive Surgery & Perioperative Chemotherapy for Peritoneal Surface Malignancy. Textbook and Video Atlas. Cine-Med Publishing: Woodbury, CT, 2012, 1-30.

[40] Ozols, RF; Young, RC; Speyer, JL; et al. Phase I and pharmacologic studies of adriamycin administered intraperitoneally to patients with ovarian cancer. *Cancer Res*, 1982, 42, 4265-4269.

[41] Rossi, CR; Foletto, M; Mocellin, S; et al. Hyperthermic intraoperative intraperitoneal chemotherapy with cisplatin and doxorubicin in patients who undergo cytoreductive surgery for peritoneal carcinomatosis and sarcomatosis. Phase I study. *Cancer*, 2002, 94, 492-499.

[42] Sugarbaker, PH; Van der Speeten, K; Stuart, OA; Chang, D. Impact of surgical and clinical factors on the pharmacology of intraperitoneal doxorubicin in 145 patients with peritoneal carcinomatosis. *Eur J Surg Oncol*, 2011, 37, 719-726.

[43] Van der Speeten, K; Stuart, OA; Sugarbaker, PH. A pharmacologic analysis of intraoperative intracavitary cancer chemotherapy with doxorubicin. *Cancer Chemother Pharmacol*, 2009, 63(5), 799-805.

[44] Sugarbaker, PH; Jacquet, P; Stephens, AD; Stuart, OA; Averbach, AM. Comparison of covered versus closed technique for heated intraoperative intraperitoneal chemotherapy for peritoneal carcinomatosis from gastrointestinal cancer. (In) Abe O, Inokuchi K, Takasaki K (eds); XXX World Congress of the International College of Surgeons. Monduzzi Editore: Bologna, 1996, 389-393.

In: Doxorubicin
Editor: Melinda Pache
ISBN: 978-1-63117-233-5

Chapter 2

PRECLINICAL CHARACTERIZATION OF THE DRUG-DELIVERY DEVICE DCBEADS™ FOR TRANSARTERIAL CHEMOEMBOLIZATION OF DOXORUBICIN AND NEMORUBICIN, A METHOXY-MORPHOLINYL DERIVATIVE

***Francesco Fiore*[1], *Olga Valota*[2], *Dario Ballinari*[2], *Federico Riccardi Sirtori*[2], *Maristella Colombo*[2], *Michela D'Antò*[1], *Cristina Geroni*[2] *and Paolo Cappella*[2*]**

[1]National Cancer Institute G. Pascale Fondation, Napoli, Italy
[2]Drug Discovery Oncology, Nerviano Medical Sciences srl, Nerviano, Italy

ABSTRACT

Hepatocellular carcinoma (HCC) represents a challenging malignancy of worldwide relevance and it is one of the most common causes of cancer-related death globally. Therapies that offer a high rate of responses in HCC include surgical resection, transplantation and percutaneous ablation. Among the non-curative therapies, transarterial chemoembolization (TACE) is a minimally invasive approach for

---

* paolo.cappella@nervianoms.com.

palliative treatment of liver tumours combining embolization and chemotherapeutic effects and employed as an adjunctive therapy to liver resection or as a bridge to liver transplantation, as well as prior to radiofrequency ablation. Conventional TACE typically involves the injection of chemotherapeutic agents such as doxorubicin (DX), with lipiodol with or without embolic agent, into the branch of the hepatic artery that feeds the tumor lesion.

Being HCCs poorly responsive tumors, new strategies such as the use of novel drug delivery systems capable of a sustained intra-tumoral release of an anticancer agent with minimal host toxicity warrant investigation. Nemorubicin (PNU-152243A, methoxymorpholinyl DX) is a derivative of DX, 70-times more potent than DX that, although structurally similar, differs substantially for the mechanism of action, the pattern of resistance and metabolism. Unlike DX, nemorubicin is not sensitive to the expression of membrane glycoproteins important for the efflux of the drug and then exceeds the MDR1 resistance often observable with DX derivatives. Based on drug metabolism studies and the high therapeutic response rate observed in HCC patients receiving IHA administration of the drug during clinical trials, nemorubicin may be considered a good choice for locoregional treatment of HCC.

DCBeads™ are spherical microparticles, formulated into beads of varying size, which the presence of anionic charges enables them to interact with positively charged drugs, such as DX. Microspheres can both target their drug cargo by physical trapping in blood vessels and sustain the action of a therapeutic agent through controlled in situ release and clinical studies have showed that TACE with DCBeads™ loaded with DX is an effective and safe procedure in the treatment of HCC patients

The present study was undertaken to obtain preclinical data on the possible use of nemorubicin-loaded DCBeads™ for tumor chemotherapy and embolization. The main objectives of this study were the evaluation of the kinetics of loading and release of nemorubicin into and from DCBeads™, the assessment of the size and spherical shape of DCBeads™ upon nemorubicin loading, and the cytotoxic activity of the released nemorubicin towards tumor cells, in comparison with DX.

Nemorubicin loading into DCBeads™ was fast with a loading rate similar to DX. Conversely, DX showed a slower kinetic and a relevant amount of unreleased (97%) compound. The released drugs maintained the same antiproliferative activities on tumor cells that the unloaded drugs. Morphometric analysis of DCBeads™ during loading and release studies showed that, unlike DX, nemorubicin did not alter the physical characteristics of microspheres that maintain their shape and volume thus preserving their foreseen embolic potential. DCBeads™ are easily loaded with nemorubicin at clinically applicable dosages; loading and elution data support considering nemorubicin a suitable drug for TACE through microspheres.

Keywords: DCBeads™, hepatocellular carcinoma, HCC, doxorubicin, Nemorubicin, multi drug resistance

INTRODUCTION

Hepatocellular carcinoma (HCC) represents a challenging malignancy of worldwide relevance. It is one of the most common causes of cancer-related death globally [1,2].

The multikinase inhibitor Sorafenib has shown survival benefits in patients with HCC and represents a breakthrough in the management of this disease [3]. Sorafenib was approved in late 2007 for HCC based on phase III trial results [SHARP] in which patients with advanced HCC, which did not receive prior systemic therapy, were evaluated and randomized to receive either sorafenib or placebo.

The trial was stopped showing a statistically significant advantage for sorafenib over placebo for overall survival. This study represents a landmark in the treatment of HCC, since it was the first time that a systemic agent improved overall survival in advanced HCC. It thereby set the standard for the first-line treatment of the disease [4].

Despite the positive results of improved overall survival obtained in the SHARP study, the benefits remain limited and the need for additional therapies that further improve efficacy for patients with HCC continue to be challenging.

Therapies that offer a high rate of responses in HCC include surgical resection, transplantation and percutaneous ablation. Among the non-curative therapies, transarterial chemoembolization (TACE) was considered of value and recommended in 2005 by the AASLD Practice Guideline [5] as first line non-curative therapy in non-surgical patients with large-multifocal HCC and no vascular invasion or extra-hepatic spread [6].

TACE is a minimally invasive approach for palliative treatment of liver tumours combining embolization and chemotherapeutic effects and employed as an adjunctive therapy to liver resection or as a bridge to liver transplantation, as well as prior to radiofrequency ablation [7,8]. Conventional TACE typically involves the injection of chemotherapeutic agents such as doxorubicin (DX), with lipiodol with or without embolic agent, into the branch of the hepatic artery that feeds the tumor lesion [4,5].

Although it has been reported that TACE in HCC patients showed better survival benefits compared to best supportive care [3], there is no consensus about the best anticancer agent to be applied, the best technique and the optimal schedule of treatment.

In addition, being HCCs poorly responsive tumors, new strategies such as the use of novel drug delivery systems capable of a sustained intra-tumoral release of an anticancer agent with minimal host toxicity warrant investigation. Nemorubicin (nemorubicin hydrochloride, PNU-152243A) is a non-conventional anthracycline, currently in Phase II clinical evaluation in HCC patients, able to overcome several mechanisms of tumor drug resistance and with minimal cardiotoxicity then DX.

Based on drug metabolism studies demonstrating hepatic conversion of nemorubicin to a more cytotoxic species [27] and the high therapeutic response rate observed in HCC patients receiving IHA administration of the drug during phase I and II trials [9,10,10,12], nemorubicin may be considered a good choice for locoregional treatment of HCC.

DCBeads™ are spherical microparticles composed by polyvinyl alcohol (PVA) hydrogel-modified by hydrophilic ionic monomer 2-acrylamido-2-methylpropanesulphonate sodium salts and formulated into beads of varying size from 100-900 μm.

The presence of negative anionic charges in the sulphonate groups of DCBeads™ enables them to interact with positively-charged drugs, such as DX. DX has shown significative acidic due to protonated amine on sugar moiety amine (DX, pKa 9.1) or methoxymorpholine (nemorubicin, pKa 5.6) residues resulting compatible to interaction to sulphonated groups on negative charged polymer (Figure 1).

Being solid porous particles, microspheres can both target their drug cargo by physical trapping in blood vessels (chemoembolization), and sustain the action of a therapeutic agent through controlled in situ release. Clinical study have showed that TACE with DCBeads™ loaded with DX is an effective and safe procedure in the treatment of HCC patients [12,16,17].

The present study was undertaken to obtain preliminary data on the possible use of nemorubicin-loaded DCBeads™ for tumor chemotherapy and embolization.

The main objectives of this study were the evaluation of the kinetics of loading and release of nemorubicin into and from DCBeads™, the assessment of the size and spherical shape of DCBeads™ upon nemorubicin loading, and the cytotoxic activity of the released nemorubicin towards tumor cells. All studies were performed in comparison with DX.

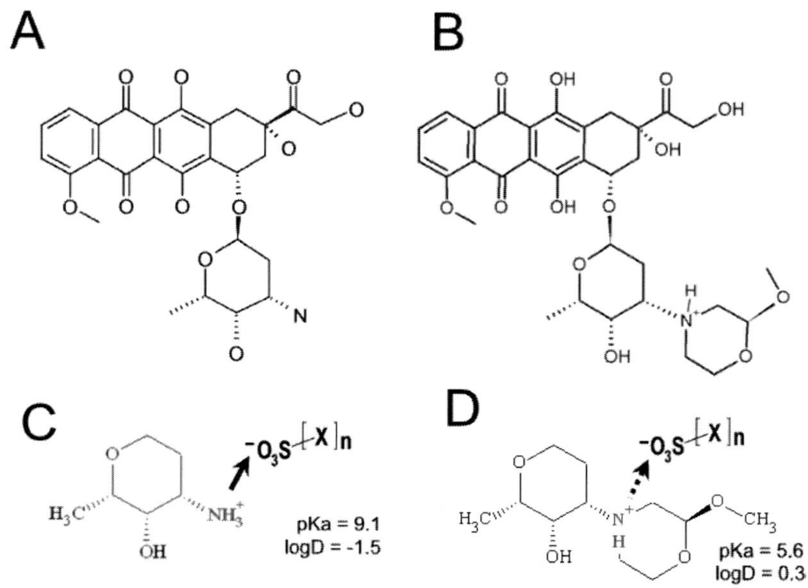

Figure 1. Comparison with different physical and chemical characteristics for the members of anthracyclins class, A, Doxorubicin (DX), B, Nemorubicin described in this chapter and relative binding with 2-methylpropanesulphonate residues in DCBeads™ consistent to basicity (pKa) and lipofilicity (logD) for C, DX and D, Nemorubicin.

Preclinical Development of DCBeads™ Loaded with Nemorubicin in Comparison to DX

Loading Efficiency and Elution Kinetics

DCBeads™ (size range 100-300 μm) were loaded with nemorubicin (0.5, 1 and 2 mg/ml, final concentration) in agreement with of the doses applied in the clinical setting [10]. DX was tested in parallel, at the concentration of 25 mg/ml, as reported in the DCBeads™ protocol for clinical use [14] and at 1 mg/ml in order to make a cross-comparison with nemorubicin concentrations.

DCBeads™ microspheres were loaded with the drug substance applying the standard protocol used also in the clinical setting.

DCBeads™ (100-300μm diameter) were exposed to drugs in water at 37°C. At the end of loading time, nemorubicin-DCBeads™ and DX-DCBeads™ were washed in water and supernatants were collected for drug quantification (as reported in Materials and Methods).

As reported (Table 1) in a non-ionic solution (water), the loading efficiency of nemorubicin by DCBeads™ after 1 and 2h incubation was more than 99% at all tested doses. Similar results were obtained with DX. Microscopic analysis showed that the loading kinetic of nemorubicin and DX is very quick and dose-dependent [20].

DCBeads™ loaded (1h incubation) with nemorubicin (1mg/ml) or DX (1 and 25mg/ml) were incubated in PBS or human plasma at 37°C for the evaluation of the kinetic of drug-elution at the following time points: 1, 24, 48, 72, 96, 120, 144h. As control, the elution rate of both drugs was tested in water.

Table 1. Loading efficiency of DCBeads™ exposed to nemorubicin or DX

Drug	Dose (mg drug /ml DCBeads™)	Drug loading (%) (1 h incubation)
Nemorubicin	0.5	99.4
	1	99.5
	2	99.8
DX	1	99.7
	25	99.8

Table 2. Elution-rate of nemorubicin and DX after 24 and 144h incubation in ionic and non-ionic media

Drug	DCBeads™ incubated with mg/ml	Elution rate (%)[1]			
		Water 24h	PBS 24h	PBS 144h	Plasma 144h
Nemorubicin	1	0.4	51.4	85	94
DX	1	0.1	1.4	60	not tested
	25	0.3	1.1	4	3.4

In Table 2 we showed that the drug released in water was minimal being only the 0.4% of the loaded nemorubicin (1mg/ml) and 0.1 and 0.3% of the loaded DX (1 and 25mg/ml, respectively).

DCBeads™ (100-300μm diameter) were exposed to drugs 1h in water at 37°C. At the end of loading time drug-loaded microspheres were incubated in water (non-ionic media), PBS and human plasma (ionic media). Samples of the media were collected at different times up to 144h.[1)] % of drug in the media versus the total loaded drug. Mean of two independent experiments.

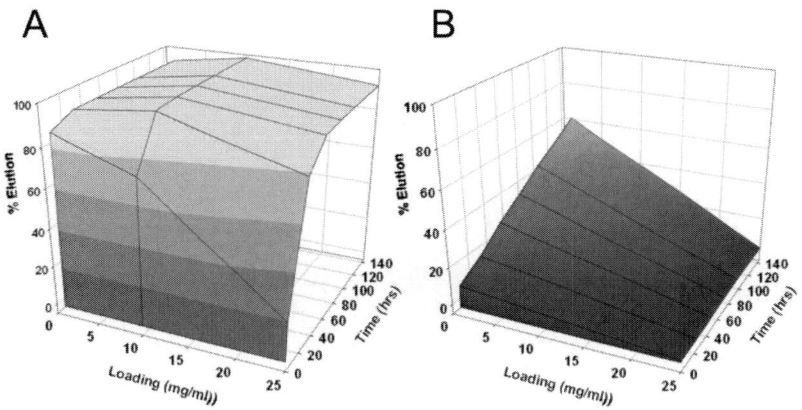

Figure 2. Nemorubicin (A) and DX (B): dose-dependence cumulative elution (%).

Nemorubicin (A) and DX (B): dose-dependence cumulative elution. Drug amounts were calculated according determination by LC/MS analysis and eluted volumes. Cumulative elutions were calculated based on loading at different concentration of nemorubicin and DX in DCBeads™ and percentages values were ratios between cumulative eluted drugs divided by total loading drugs.

Into isotonic media (PBS) the amount of released nemorubicin was very high 51% and 85% at 24 and 144h, respectively. Conversely, the delivery of DX, at the dose used in clinic of 25 mg/ml, was lower (1.1% and 4% at 24 and 144h, respectively) than nemorubicin showing that a higher amount of DX remains entrapped into DCBeads™. Similar results were obtained in human plasma with 94% and 4% of nemorubicin or DX, respectively, released at time 144h (Table 2).

Figure 2 reported the kinetics of drug-release in PBS. Nemorubicin (1mg/ml) was completely released in 96h while DX (1mg/ml) was still detectable at 144h. The elution-rate at higher doses of nemorubicin (up to 25 mg/ml loading) showed that nemorubicin delivering was higher and faster than DX independently from the dose.

Morphometric Analysis

The size and spherical shape of DCBeads™ were analyzed during both the loading and the release processes of nemorubicin and DX up to 144h.

Table 3. Size of DCBeads™ microspheres after nemorubicin or DX - loading and at different drug elution times in PBS

		Control		Nemorubicin		DX	
		DCBeads™ in PBS	Calibration beads	1 mg drug/ml DCBeads™	25 mg drug/ml DCBeads™	1 mg drug/ml DCBeads™	25 mg drug/ml DCBeads™
	Time (h)	Mean (Øµm ± SD)	Mean (Øµm ± SD)	Mean (Øµm ± SD)	Mean (Øµm ± SD)	Mean (Øµm ± SD)	Mean (Øµm ± SD)
Loading	1	217 ± 58	76 ± 12	248 ± 70 p=0.07	217 ± 53 p=0.03	223 ± 68 p=0.07	160 ± 73 p=0.01
Elution	1	274± 47	73 ± 11	258 ± 64 p=0.71			94 ± 27 p<0.0001
	24	271 ± 64	86 ± 16	284 ± 62 p=0.56			98 ± 27 p<0.0001
	48	260 ± 47	80 ± 15	251 ± 41 p=0.41			106 ± 34 p<0.0001
	72	261 ± 36	86 ± 17	244 ± 59 p=0.12			116 ± 32 p<0.0001
	96	250 ± 32	89 ± 13	222 ± 41 p=0.07			126 ± 43 p<0.0001
	144	235 ± 53	87 ± 15	232 ± 39 p=0.97	242 ± 12 p=0.67	188 ± 77 p=0.002	169 ± 53 p<0.0001

As shown in Table 3 both the loading and release of nemorubicin (1 mg/ml) did not interfere with the size of DCBeads™; the size range was 248 ± 70 and 232 ± 39 for nemorubicin and 217 ± 58 and 235 ± 53 for controls after 1h loading and 6 days release, respectively. Conversely, DCBeads™ treated with DX showed a decreased size (160 ± 73 and 169 ± 53 after 1h loading and

6 days release, respectively) compared to controls. In addition DX-loaded DC Beads showed high heterogeneity [supplementary details in ref 20].

These results correlate with the microscope evaluation that showed that unlike DCBeads™ loaded with DX that are very small, nemorubicin-DC Beads maintained the same size as the unloaded ones (Figure 3).

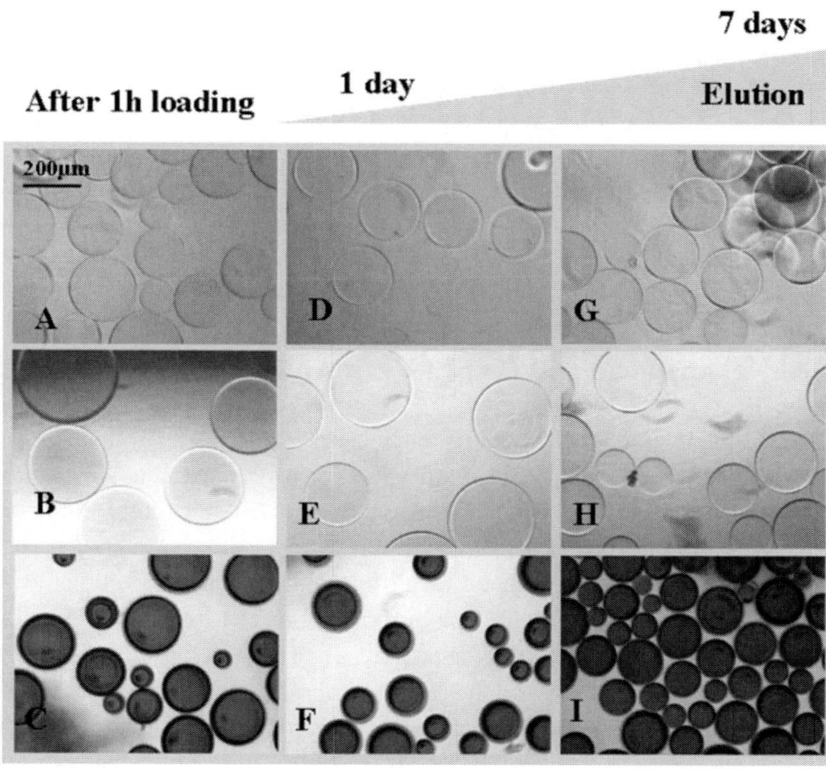

Figure 3. Appearance of DCBeads^{TM} loaded with nemorubicin (1mg/ml) or DX (25 mg/ml).

These results were correlate with the microscope evaluation that showed that nemorubicin-loaded DCBeads™ loaded with DX that are very small, nemorubicin-DC Beads maintained the same size as the unloaded ones. No aggregation was observed for loaded or unloaded microspheres. These features may offer a great advantage for the administration of the nemorubicin formulation in microspheres to obtain a proper embolization effect.

Morphometric analysis of loaded DCBeads™s loaded with nemorubicin or DX by Image Pro Plus™ (Media Cybernatics) and 108μm PMMA beads were used for size calibration. Appearance was determined by a DM IRB (Leica) microscope equipped with an Evolution MP Color CCD Camera (Media Cybernatics). For size experiments 20µl of DCBeads™ with or without drug were placed in 200µl distillated water into 48-wells plate (Corning) and observed at 5x/0.12 magnification. Morphometric analysis was done by Image Pro Plus™ (Media Cybernatics) and 108µm PMMA beads (Bangs Laboratories) were used for size calibration. Statistical analysis was performed by SigmaPlot 10.0.

Pictures showed microscope examination of DCBeads™ microspheres at 1 h loading with nemorubicin at 1mg/ml and DX 25mg/ml and after 1 and 6 days of drug elution in phosphate buffer solution. A-D-G) controls, B-E-H) nemorubicin at 1mg/ml and C-F-I) DX at 25mg/ml at 1hour loading and after 1 and 7 days of drug elution Pictures were performed using a DM IRB microscope equipped with a color CCD Camera (5x/0.12 magnification) [20].

Eluted Nemorubicin and DX: In Vitro Antiproliferative Activity

Nemorubicin and DX fractions eluted from DCBeads™ (loaded with nemorubicin 1mg/ml or DX 25 mg/ml) were tested in vitro against human mammary carcinoma cells MCF-7 and on human hepatocellular carcinoma (HepG2) cell lines (Table 4).

Cells were treated for 72 h by raise dilutions of elution fractions or for standard (1) with a fresh prepared solution. At the end of treatment, cells were processed as reported in Materials and Methods. The dose inhibiting the 50% of cell growth (IC_{50}) was calculated using sigmoidal interpolation curve. (2) R.I. = Resistance Index value obtained by comparing the IC_{50} on resistant (MCF-7/DX) and sensitive (MCF7) cells. (3) N/A not applicable. (4) Data adapted from [21]. Experiments were carried out at least twice. Mean, coefficient of variation (CV %) and Pearson test is analyzed by Graph Pad Prism 5.

Nemorubicin is effective at concentrations seven times higher than DX on MCF-7 cells (IC_{50} 12 and 89 nM, respectively) and eight times higher than DX on HepG2 cells (IC_{50} 9 and 76nM, respectively). In addition, nemorubicin overcomes DX resistance being effective on MCF-7/DX cells (R.I. 1.3) high resistant to DX [R.I. 123, ref. 21]. The concentrations of nemorubicin and DX present in the eluted fractions are as effective as standards up to release time of 96h in all cell lines tested and nemorubicin maintains its activity against DX resistant cells. These results are well correlated with the kinetic of drug release.

Table 4. Anti proliferative activity (IC_{50}) and capability for maintaining activity (F) of nemorubicin and DX in eluted fractions from drug-loaded DCBeads™ for nemorubicin or DX loaded in DCBeads™ microspheres

	Nemorubicin				DX			
Time (h)	MCF-7 IC_{50} (nM ± SE)	MCF-7/DX IC_{50} (nM ± SE)	R.I.	HepG2 IC_{50} (nM ± SE)	MCF-7 IC_{50} (nM ± SE)	MCF-7/DX IC_{50} (nM ± SE)	R.I.	HepG2 IC_{50} (nM ± SE)
IS	**12 ± 5** **19(4)**	**18 ± 5** **25(4)**	**1.1** **1.3(4)**	**9 ± 2**	**89 ± 35** **19(4)**	**>2,500** **2150(4)**	**>28** **123(4)**	**76 ± 31**
0 (1)	20 ± 7	41 ± 3	2.1	15 ± 4	69± 20	>2500	>36	50 ± 14
1	17 ± 5	30 ± 5	1.7	13 ± 2	64 ± 35	>2500		69 ± 31
24	7 ± 5	8 ± 5	1.4	8 ± 3	106 ± 35	>2500		103 ± 40
48	15 ± 2	17 ± 2	1.4	9 ± 2	159 ± 47	>2500		147 ± 61
72	4 ± 4	17 ± 2	1.2	7 ± 2	188 ± 72	>2500		189 ± 73
96	9 ± 1	6 ± 2	1.2	5 ± 1	207 ± 84	>2500		196 ± 80
144	13± 4	16 ± 2	1.5	11 ± 2	233 ± 91	>2500		241 ± 84
mean	**13± 2**	**21 ± 5**		**11± 2**	**147± 26**	**>2500**		**142± 27**
CV%	41	33		36	44	N/A (3)		48
Pearson r	-0.22	-0.32		-0.24	0.93	N/A (3)		0.96
F	0.9± 0.2	0.7 ± 0.2		0.8± 0.2	1.2± 0.2	N/A (3)		2.3± 0.4

Cells were treated for 72 h by raise dilutions of free solutions or for standard (1) with a fresh prepared solution (IS). At the end of treatment, cells were processed as reported in Materials and Methods. The dose inhibiting the 50% of cell growth (IC_{50}) was calculated using sigmoidal interpolation curve. (2) R.I. = Resistance Index value obtained by comparing the IC_{50} on resistant (MCF-7/DX) and sensitive (MCF7) cells. (3) NA not applicable. (4) Data adapted from [21] Experiments were carried out at least twice. Mean, coefficient of variation (CV %) and Pearson test is analyzed by Graph Pad Prism 5.

Since a drug delivery device should exerts a protective effect towards the chemical stability of nemorubicin, we compared IC50 from eluted fraction and free drugs in PBS solutions maintained in same experimental conditions (from

1h to 144h) with IC50 from internal standard (IS) and resulting ratios (F parameter) are shown in Table 4. All data from free solutions were shown in Table 5.

Table 5. Anti proliferative activity (IC_{50}) and capability for maintaining activity (F) of nemorubicin and DX in free solutions for nemorubicin or DX drugs

	Nemorubicin				DX			
Time (h)	MCF-7 IC_{50} (nM ± SE)	MCF-7/DX IC_{50} (nM ± SE)	R.I.	HepG2 IC_{50} (nM ± SE)	MCF-7 IC_{50} (nM ± SE)	MCF-7/DX IC_{50} (nM ± SE)	R.I.	HepG2 IC_{50} (nM ± SE)
IS	**12 ± 5** **19**[(4)]	**18 ± 5** **25**[(4)]	**1.1** **1.3**[(4)]	**9 ± 2**	**89 ± 35** **19**[(4)]	**>2,500** **2150**[(4)]	**>28** **123**[(4)]	**76 ± 31**
0 (1)	20 ± 5	37 ± 4	1.5	12 ± 2	90 ± 31	>2500	>28	66 ± 20
1	28 ± 8	50 ± 4	1.7	15 ± 4	71 ± 20	>2500		50 ± 14
24	22 ± 6	38 ± 7	1.7	14 ± 3	114 ± 31	>2500		101 ± 19
48	26 ± 7	40 ± 5	1.5	16 ± 4	172 ± 49	>2500		198 ± 36
72	27 ± 7	42 ± 4	1.6	17 ± 4	243 ± 63	>2500		316 ± 51
96	26 ± 6	38 ± 1	1.5	17 ± 4	381 ± 72	>2500		534 ± 93
144	29 ± 3	45 ± 2		20 ± 3	481 ± 27	>2500		621 ± 47
mean	**24 ± 2**	**39 ± 4**		**15 ± 2**	**222 ± 60**	**>2500**		**271 ± 87**
CV%	19	26		13	69	N/A (3)		81
Pearson r	0.25	0.13		-0.11	0.98	N/A (3)		0.97
F	2.2 ± 0.3	2.1 ± 0.4		1.7 ± 0.3	1.8 ± 0.7	N/A (3)		4.4 ± 1.4

Eluted nemorubicin is found more stable (F closed to 1) than free nemorubicin in PBS (F above to 2) and in general comparing to DX (from DCBeads™ eluted and free solution, F = 1.8 and 3.1 respectively). Moreover, is observed a linear association between anti proliferative activity decreasing and elution time for DX (Pearson r closed to 1 for DX), whereas for nemorubicin, the correlation is not meaningful.

Nemorubicin and DX elution from DCBeads™ were investigated with different media (water, PBS and human plasma) and with different volume of beads and drug solution. According to the experimental data, nemorubicin and DX prove to be adequately stable over the considered time.

CONCLUSION

Transcatheter arterial chemoembolisation (TACE) is a standard therapy in the treatment of hepatocellular carcinoma (HCC) patients in intermediate stage (according to BCLC) but still there is no consensus about the optimal chemotherapeutic and embolic agent. Microspheres made from a compressible polyvinyl alcohol hydrogel are a new embolic product that is capable of being loaded with anticancer drugs before administration in TACE procedure. The potential benefits of such microspheres are considerable because a sustainable release of chemotherapy over time could have a greater impact on tumor kill.

Critical determinants in defining the pharmacological activity of TACE performed with microspheres are the: firstly, preservation of the native conformation (size and spherical shape) for an appropriate occlusion of the lumen of the liver vessels and avoiding distal embolization; secondly, loading rate of the chemotherapeutic agents to guarantee the administration of therapeutic doses; thirdly release rate of the loaded drug to allow high intra-tumor drug concentrations for a sufficient period of time and finally complete release of the active agent to avoid unexpected side effects. Nemorubicin loading, at all clinically useful concentrations resulted in an unchanged average size of the microspheres. This allows an accurate embolization of tumour vessels. Conversely, commercial microspheres loaded with DX have a decrease in the average size; this can impact the accuracy of the drug release in the targeted region, can reduce the efficacy against tumour, and may increase the risk of complications. In particular, the composition containing nemorubicin bound to microspheres preserves the native conformation of the microspheres (in terms of size and spherical shape) and guarantees the appropriate occlusion of the lumen of the liver vessel, avoiding distal embolization (e.g., pulmonary and/or cerebral embolization).

These unique features of the nemorubicin/microspheres loaded formulation are evident when the data herein are compared to the one described in the literature article of Lewis cited above [15], where the loading of DX in the DCBeads™ not only is dose dependant, but also induce a severe shrinkage of the DC beads™ and influence the release rate kinetic of the drug itself from the delivery system both in vitro and in vivo. DCBeads™ containing nemorubicin bound to microspheres allowed a fast loading (1h incubation) and a loading rate of nemorubicin hydrochloride into the microspheres (>99%) could be able to guarantee an easy administration of therapeutic doses of nemorubicin hydrochloride to patients.

Our study support evidences that nemorubicin and microspheres formulation was more chemically stable than the active drug substance per se while administered as locoregional therapy and that the microspheres system exerts a protective effect towards the chemical stability of nemorubicin, thus allowing the release in a controlled and sustained matter exclusively of the active moiety. DX dissolved in PBS media, kept at experimental condition, was found less active than internal standard since was degradated in inactive compounds such as Henry's acid [22,23]. Interestingly, for nemorubicin no degradation products were found and drug remain active up to 144 h.

Although structurally related to anthracycline derivative DX, nemorubicin (Figure 3), has shown a completely different mechanism of action since not cardiotoxic at optimal antitumor doses retaining antitumor activity in various resistant tumor models. In vivo evidences shown that nemorubicin is 80–120 times more potent than doxorubicin [21,24]. In contrast, its in-vitro cytotoxicity is only eight and two times greater than that of doxorubicin toward cultured drug sensitive tumor cells and hematopoietic progenitor cells, respectively [25,26]. Various studies have also shown that incubation of nemorubicin and isolated liver microsomes results in marked enhancement of potency toward cultured tumor cells, suggesting that nemorubicin is converted to a much more cytotoxic metabolites by CYP3A enzyme subfamily. Moreover a further study established that nemorubicin is converted by human liver microsomes to a major metabolite found to be 700–2400 times more potent than nemorubicin toward cultured human tumor cells, and exhibited significant efficacy in *in vivo* tumor models [27]. Conversely, DX was metabolized in less active products and excreted primarily through the hepatobiliary route [28,29,30] resulting in a reduced antitumor activity. Since CYP3A4 expression has been reported also in a broad range of human tumours, including colon rectal cancer [30], DCBeads™ containing nemorubicin could be explored for treatment of those tumours resistant to irinotecan, currently used in TACE for CRC, its activity is decreased by CYP3A4 metabolism [14,32].

The concentrations of nemorubicin present in the eluted fractions are as effective as standards up to release time of 144h in all cell lines tested and nemorubicin maintains its activity against DX resistant cells. Recent studies has determined that HCC is hierarchically organized and originated from cancer stem cells (CSCs) for which CD133+ and CD13+ precursors constitute the most immature stages [33,34]. Since CSCs are able to evade conventional therapies including DX due to high expression levels of specific MDR transporters, nemorubicin (and active metabolites) could circumvent anthracyclins debacle against tumour-initiating cells, expressing multidrug resistance [35,36].

The present study was designed to evaluate the embolic profile and in vitro cytotoxic activity of microspheres (DCBeads™) loaded with nemorubicin, an investigational anticancer agent whose intra-hepatic artery (IHA) administration was recently found to be well tolerated and effective in intermediate and advanced stage multiple HCC.

Elution experiments demonstrated that nemorubicin is released from drug-loaded DCBeads™ into isotonic medium and human plasma faster and in a higher amount than its parent drug, doxorubicin (DX). The released nemorubicin shows a cytotoxic activity towards human tumor cell lines comparable to that of fresh solutions of the drug. In addition, unlike with DX, loading of nemorubicin does not alter the shape and volume of DCBeads™, thus preserving their embolic properties.

Collectively these data suggest that nemorubicin-loaded DCBeads™ might represent a promising drug delivery system for a safe and effective treatment of HCC patients with TACE, thus deserving further studies for therapeutic potential.

MATERIALS AND METHODS

Chemicals

Nemorubicin hydrochloride (nemorubicin, PNU-152243A) and doxorubicin (DX) were purchased from Nerviano Medical Sciences, Nerviano Italy. DCBeads™ as drug delivery emboliation system (Biocompatibles UK Ltd., Farnham, UK, Ref. DC2V103) were used in the size range of 100-300µm. DC Beads™ is a drug delivery embolization system for use in TACE receiving CE mark approval in 2003. Sterile distilled water was used as vehicle for loading studies with both drugs. Other vehicles used included phosphate buffered saline pH 7.4 (PBS) (Invitrogen) and human plasma from healthy donors. All solvents and reagents used for LC/MS analysis were purchased from Sigma-Aldrich.

Nemorubicin and DX Loading and Release Kinetics by DCBeads™

Drug-eluting DCBeads™ are available in the size range 100-1000µm, here microspheres of 100-300µm diameters were used, as this size-range is the most suitable for TACE in the treatment of HCC [14].

As reported in the loading procedure (Biocompatibles guide-lines), the packing solution was removed and DCBeads™ were conditioned in water than nemorubicin (0.1, 0.5, 1 and 2 mg/ml) or DX (1 and 25 mg/ml) solutions in water were added. The mixture drug-DCBeads™ was roller-mixed gently and kept at 37°C up to 2 h. At the end of the incubation time, drug-loaded DCBeads™ were washed in water and supernatants were collected for drug quantification. The loading of nemorubicin and DX was calculated by measuring by LC/MS analysis versus a standard curve of nemorubicin or DX, the remaining drug concentration in solution over time.

Loading efficiency was calculated as: Loading Efficiency (%) = 100 x (initial drug amount – residual drug in the supernatant) / initial drug amount.

Nemorubicin and DX elution was evaluated by the incubation of drug-loaded DCBeads™ in PBS (pH 7.4) or in human plasma. At different elution time, supernatant was collected, filtered by 70μm nylon filcon filter (BD Biosciences) to avoid any carry-over contaminations and stored at –20°C.

For dose dependence cumulative elution studies, drug amount eluted at time was calculated as: % elution = total volume from eluted (in PBS) + washing fractions (in water) x [concentration] / loading amount x 100.

Quantitative Determination of Nemorubicin and DX by LC/MS Analysis

Nemorubicin and DX were measured by HPLC on a Phenomenex Gemini Phenyl (4.6 x 50 mm, 3μm) column using a Surveyor HPLC system (Thermo Electron Corporation) equipped with a PDA detector and Finnigan MAT LCQ Deca XP ion trap mass spectrometer, equipped with an electrospray (ESI) ion source. Mobile phase A was an acetate buffer 40 mM and phase B was acetate buffer 400 mM : acetonitrile 1:9 (v:v).

The following conditions were used: a gradient from 95 to 20% A in 7 min and held at 20% A for 2 min; UV detection at 480 nm; a flow rate of 1 ml/min; an injection volume of 20 μL; full scan, mass range from 50 to 1000 amu. Sample extraction procedure for human plasma involved a solid phase extraction of DX and nemorubicin from plasma using Waters Oasis HLB extraction cartridges with the procedure previously described [18].

Retention times (4.99 for DX and 6.2 min for nemorubicin, Figure 4) are given in minutes at 254, 480 nm and 580nm. The linearity of the response of the LC/MS method for nemorubicin and DX was determined with different standard solutions over the concentration up to 400μM.

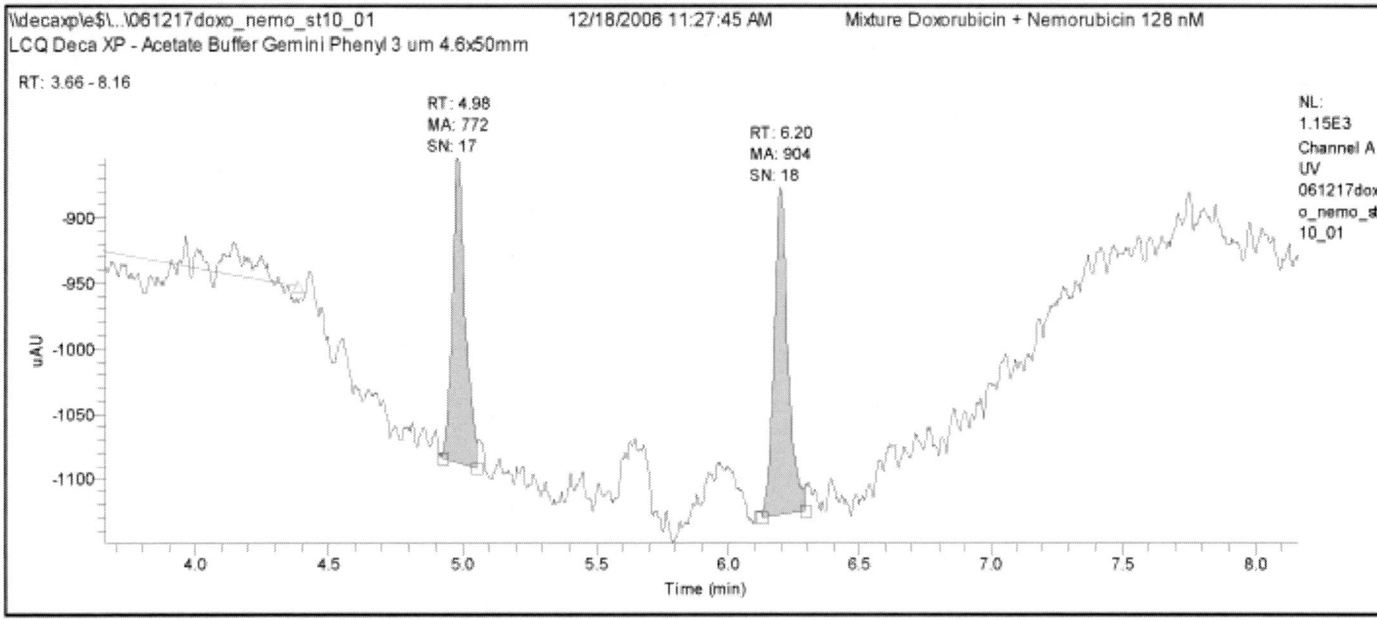

Figure 4. Typical LC chromatogram for DX and Nemorubicin detection for method sensitivity studies: limit of detection for Doxorubicin (rt 4.99) and Nemorubicin (rt 6.20).

According to the S/N ratio criterion, the experimentally achieved detection limit was 0.128 μM. The stability of the stock solutions 1 mg/ml were evaluated during the elution experiment (Table 5). Aliquots of the stock solutions 1 mg/ml (stored at 37°C) were collected at the same time of the samples coming from beads and then stored at –20°C prior analysis.

Morphometric Analysis of DCBeads™

Size and appearance of DCBeads™ with and without drug were monitored during loading and elution kinetics. Appearance was determinated by a DM IRB (Leica) microscope equipped with an Evolution MP Color CCD Camera (Media Cybernatics). For size experiments 20μl of DCBeads™ with or without drug were placed in 200μl distillated water into 48-wells plate (Corning) and observed at 5x/0.12 magnification. Morphometric analysis was done by Image Pro Plus™ (Media Cybernatics) and 108μm PMMA beads (Bangs Laboratories) were used for size calibration (Figure 5). Statistical analysis was performed by SigmaPlot 10.0 (SyStat Software).

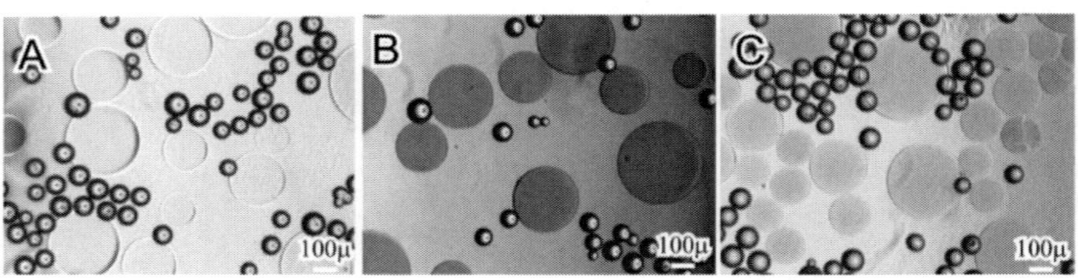

Figure 5. Diameter quantification of DCbeads™ unloaded (A), DX 25 mg/ml (B) or Nemorubicin (C) in comparison to 108μm PMMA beads used as internal calibrator.

In Vitro Antiproliferative Activity on Tumor Cells

The growth inhibition activity of drugs eluted in the collected fractions was tested on exponentially growing human mammary adenocarcinoma cells (MCF7) and on its DX-resistant subclones (MCF7/DX) and on human hepatocellular carcinoma (HepG2) cell lines (European Collection of Cell Cultures). Cells were grown in E-MEM/Glutamax medium (Invitrogen), containing 10% FBS (EuroClone) and 1% NEAA (Invitrogen) and maintained at 37°C in 5% CO2. Cells were authenticated by assessing short tandem repeats with AmpF/STR identifiler (Applied Biosystems).

For testing the antiproliferative activity, cells were seeded into 96 plates (Corning) at 5,000 /cm2 in appropriate medium. After 24 hours, cells were treated in duplicate with serial dilutions of DX or nemorubicin, and 72 hours later, viable cell number was assessed using the CellTiter-Glo Assay (Promega) and plates were read by Envision luminometer (PerkinElmer) [19]. IC50s were calculated using a Sigmoidal fitting algorithm (Assay Explorer MDL). Experiments were done independently at least twice.

The IC50 values of DX or nemorubicin in the elution medium was compared to that of fresh drug standards. All the experiments were carried out at least twice. IC50 values from eluted fraction and free solutions maintained in same experimental conditions and same time points (from 1h to 144h) are normalized by fresh internal standard IS and ratio is indicated as F parameter (fold times increase IC50 comparing IS) and results are shown in Figure 2. Mean, coefficient of variation (CV %) and Pearson test is analyzed by Graph Pad Prism 5 (Graph Pad Prism Software, San Diego, CA).

Acknowledgments

We thank Vincenzo Giansanti and Marta Durlak for critical reading.

References

[1] J Ferlay, P. Autier, M. Boniol, M. Heanue, M. Colombet, P. Boyle, Estimates of the cancer incidence and mortality in Europe in 2006, *Ann. Oncol.* 8 (2007) 581-592.

[2] Jemal, R. Siegel, E. Ward, T. Murray, J. Xu, M. J. Thun, Cancer Statistics 2007, *CA Cancer J. Clin.* 57 (2007) 43-66.

[3] J. M. Llovet, J. Bruix, Novel advancements in the management of hepatocellular carcinoma in 2008, *J. Hepatol.* 48 (2008) S20-S37.

[4] J. M. Llovet, S. Ricci, V. Mazzaferro, P. Hilgard, J. Raoul, S. Zeuzem, M. Poulin-Costello, M. Moscovici, D. Voliotis, J. Bruix, Sorafenib improves survival in advanced hepatocellular carcinoma (HCC): results of a Phase III randomized placebo-controlled trial (SHARP trial), *J. Clin. Oncol 25* (2007) LBA1.

[5] J. Bruix, M. Sherman, Management of Hepatocellular Carcinoma. AASLD Practice Guideline. *Hepat.* 42 (2005) 1208-1236.

[6] R. Miraglia, G. Pietrosi, L. Maruzzelli, I. Petridis, S. Caruso, G. Marrone, G. Mamone, G. Vizzini, A. Luca, B. Gridelli, Efficacy of transcatheter embolization/chemoembolization (TAE/TACE) for the

treatment of single hepatocellular carcinoma. *World J. Gastroenterol.* 13 (2007) 2952-2955.

[7] T. Aoki, H. Imamura, K. Hasegawa, A. Matsukura, K. Sano,Y. Sugawara, N. Kokudo, M. Makuuchi, Sequential preoperative arterial and portal venous embolizations in patients with hepatocellular carcinoma. *Arch. Surg.* 139 (2004) 766-774.

[8] J. Bruix, M. Sala, J. M. Llovet, Chemoembolization for hepatocellular carcinoma. *Gastroenterology* 127 (2004) 179-188.

[9] C. Sessa, O. Valota, C. Geroni, Ongoing Phase I and II studies of novel anthracyclines. *Cardiovasc Toxicol.* 7 (2007) 75-79.

[10] F. Fiore, C. D. Gadaleta, C. Granetto, M. Middleton, R. Sorio, R. Labianca, O. Valota, R. N. Pirotta, R. Battaglia and F. Izzo, Nemorubicin hydrochloride (nemorubicin) in combination with cisplatin (cDDP): phase I in patients(pts) with Hepatocellular Carcinoma (HCC), *J. Clin. Oncol.* (Meeting Abstracts) 26 (2008) 2572.

[11] F. Izzo, M. Grosso, M. Middleton, L. Balestreri, R. Labianca, A.M. Catino, O. Valota, B. Laffranchi, F. Fiore, Phase I study of nemorubicin hydrochloride (nemorubicin), a novel DNA-intercalator, in combination with cisplatin in patients with unresectable hepatocellular carcinoma (HCC) *Proceedings for AACR-NCI-EORTC* 2007;A 139.

[12] K. Malagari, Drug-eluting particles in the treatment of HCC: chemoembolization with doxorubicin-loaded DC Bead, *Expert Rev. Anticancer Ther.* 10 (2008) 1643-1650.

[13] T. Ronnie, P. Poon, W. K. Tso, R.W. Pang, K. K. Ng, R. Woo, K. S. Tai, S. T. Fan, A Phase I/II Trial of Chemoembolization for Hepatocellular Carcinoma Using a Novel Intra-Arterial Drug-Eluting Bead. *Clin. Gastroenterol Hepatol.* 5 (2007) 1100-1118.

[14] C. D. Gadaleta, G. Ranieri, Trans-arterial chemoembolization as a therapy for liver tumours: New clinical developments and suggestions for combination with angiogenesis inhibitors. *Crit. Rev. Oncol. Hematol.* (2011); in press.

[15] A. L. Lewis, M. V. Gonzalez, A. W. Lloyd, B. Hall, Y. Tang, S. L. Willis, S. W. Leppard, L. C. Wolfenden, R. R. Palmer, P.W. Stratford, DC bead: in vitro characterization of a drug-delivery device for transarterial chemoembolization. *J. Vasc. Interv. Radiol.* 17 (2006) 335-342.

[16] K. Malagari, K. Chatzimichael, E. Alexopoulou, A. Kelekis, B. Hall, S. Dourakis, S. Delis, A. Gouliamos, D. Kelekis, Transarterial Chemoembolization of Unresectable Hepatocellular Carcinoma with

Drug Eluting Beads: Results of an Open-Label Study of 62 Patients. *Cardiovasc Intervent Radiol.* 31 (2008) 269-280.

[17] O. Nawawi, M. N. Hazman, B. J. J. Abdullah, A. Vijayananthan, J. Manikam, S. Mahadeva, K. L. Goh, Transarterial embolisation of hepatocellular carcinoma with doxorubicin-eluting beads: single centre early experience. *Biomed. Imaging Interv. J.* 6 (2010) e7.

[18] D. Fraier, E. Frigerio, G. Brianceschi, C. A. James, LC-MS-MS determination of Nemorubicin (methoxymorpholinyldoxorubicin, PNU-152243A) and its 13-OH metabolite (PNU-155051A) in human plasma, *J. Pharm. Biomed. Anal.* 30 (2002) 377–389.

[19] F. Del Bene, M. Germani, G. De Nicolao, P. Magni, C.E. Re, D. Ballinari, M. Rocchetti, A model-based approach to the in vitro evaluation of anticancer activity. *Cancer Chemother. Pharmacol.* 63 (2009) 827-836.

[20] C. Geroni, O. Valota, A. Martini, P. Cappella, Pharmaceutical composition of the anthracyclin 2008. Patent WO/138,758. *US Patent and Trademark Office*, filled 30 april.

[21] M. Broggini, Nemorubicin. Anthracycline Chemistry and Biology II, *Top. Curr. Chem.* 283 (2008) 191-206.

[22] J. H. Beijnen, O. A. G. J. Van der Houwen, W. J. M. Underberg, Aspects of the degradation kinetics of doxorubicin in aqueous solution *Int. J. Pharm.* 32 (1986) 123-131.

[23] G. Tong, W. W. Lee, D. R. Black, D. W. Henry, Adriamycin analogs. Periodate oxidation of adriamycin *J. Med. Chem.* 19 (1976) 395–398.

[24] M. A. Sabatino, M. Marabese, M. Ganzinelli, E. Caiola, C. Geroni, M. Broggini, Down-regulation of the nucleotide excision repair gene XPG as a new mechanism of drug resistance in human and murine cancer cells *Mol Cancer.* 9 (2010) 259-259.

[25] L. Quintieri, A. Rosato, E. Napoli, F. Sola, C. Geroni, M. Floreani, P. Zanovello, In vivo antitumor activity and host toxicity of methoxymorpholinyl doxorubicin: role of cytochrome P450 3A. *Cancer Res.* 60 (2000) 3232–3238.

[26] M. Ghielmini, E. Colli, G. Bosshard, G. Pennella, C. Geroni, V. Torri, M. D'Incalci, F. Cavalli, C. Sessa. Hematotoxicity on human bone marrow- and umbilical cord blood-derived progenitor cells and in vitro therapeutic index of methoxymorpholinyldoxorubicin and its metabolites, *Cancer Chemother Pharmacol* 42 (1998) 235-40.

[27] L. Quintieri, M. Fantin, P. Palatini, S. De Martin, A. Rosato, M. Caruso, C. Geroni, M. Floreani. In vitro hepatic conversion of the anticancer

agent nemorubicin to its active metabolite PNU-159682 in mice, rats and dogs: a comparison with human liver microsomes. *Biochem. Pharmacol.* 15 (2008) 784-795.

[28] K. Mross, P. Maessen, W. J. van der Vijgh, H. Gall, E. Boven, H. M. Pinedo, Pharmacokinetics and metabolism of epidoxorubicin and doxorubicin in humans *J. Clin. Oncol.* 6 (1988) 517-526.

[29] E. Ferrazzi, J. M. Woynarowski, A. Arakali, D. E. Brenner, T. A. Beerman DNA damage and cytotoxicity induced by metabolites of anthracycline antibiotics doxorubicin and idarubicin. *Cancer Commun.* 3 (1991) 173–180.

[30] M. Binaschi, M. Bigioni, A. Cipollone, C. Rossi, C. Goso, C. A. Maggi, G. Capranico, F. Animati. Anthracyclines: selected new developments. *Curr. Med. Chem. Anticancer Agents* 1 (200) 113–130.

[31] C. Martínez, E. García-Martín, R. M. Pizarro, F. J. García-Gamito, J. A. Agúndez. Expression of paclitaxel-inactivating CYP3A activity in human colorectal cancer: implications for drug therapy. *Br. J. Cancer.* 87 (2002) 681–686.

[32] H. Lu, C. S. Chen and D. J. Waxman. Potentiation of methoxymorpholinyl doxorubicin antitumor activity by P450 3A4 gene transfer. *Cancer Gene Ther.* 16 (2009) 393–404.

[33] S. Ma, T. K. Lee, B. J. Zheng, K. W. Chan, X. Y. Guan, CD133+ HCC cancer stem cells confer chemoresistance by preferential expression of the Akt/PKB survival pathway, *Oncogene* 27 (2008) 1749-1758.

[34] N. Haraguchi, H. Ishii, K. Mimori, F. Tanaka, M. Ohkuma, H. M. Kim, H. Akita, D. Takiuchi, H. Hatano, H. Nagano, G.F. Barnard, Y. Doki, M. Mori, CD13 is a therapeutic target in human liver cancer stem cells, *J. Clin. Invest.* 120 (2010) 3326-3339.

[35] S. Ma, K. W. Chan, L. Hu, T. K. Lee, J. Y. Wo, I.O. Ng, B. J. Zheng, X. Y. Guan, Identification and characterization of tumorigenic liver cancer stem/progenitor cells. *Gastroenterology* 132 (2007) 2542-2556.

[36] Y. An, W. M. Ongkeko, Structure and function of the human breast cancer resistance protein (BCRP/ABCG2). *Curr. Drug Metab.* 11 (2010) 603-617.

In: Doxorubicin
Editor: Melinda Pache

ISBN: 978-1-63117-233-5

Chapter 3

DOXORUBICIN-INDUCED CARDIOMYOPATHY

***Xia Wang*[*1], *Wei Han*[1*], *Yan Yu*[2*], *Jinzhou Zhu*[3] and *Ruiyan Zhang*[3*]**

[1]Laboratory of Regeneromics, School of Pharmacy, Shanghai Jiao Tong University, Shanghai, China

[2]Shanghai Municipality Key Laboratory of Veterinary Biotechnology, School of Agriculture and Biology, Shanghai Jiao Tong University, Shanghai, China

[3]Department of Cardiology, Rui Jin Hospital, School of Medicine, Shanghai Jiao Tong University, Shanghai, China

ABSTRACT

Doxorubicin (DOX), an anticancer anthracycline antibiotic, is widely used in varieties of neoplastic diseases, such as leukemia, lymphomas, and solid tumors of the lung and breast. The most well known toxicity of anthracycline is its cardiac and cardiovascular toxicity. Without exception, clinical use of doxorubicin is limited by its cumulative and dose-dependent cardiomyopathy and congestive heart failure. The acute side effects of DOX treatment, such as myelosuppression, nausea, vomiting, pericarditis, myocarditis, and arrhythmia, are generally

* Corresponding authors emails: weihan@sjtu.edu.cn or yanyu@sjtu.edu.cn or ruiyanzhang@sjtu.edu.cn.

reversible and clinically manageable. As congestive heart failure is irreversible and life-threaten to patients with chronic DOX treatment, the prognosis and management of the congestive heart failure becomes critical. Several mechanisms such as free radical-dependent lipid peroxidation, mitochondrial dysfunction, calcium overload, and inhibition of membrane bound molecules have been reported for the DOX cardiotoxicity. This chapter provides an update to the pathological mechanism of DOX-induced cardiotoxicity. We also review and compare strategies in the management of DOX cardiotoxicity.

1. INTRODUCTION

Doxorubicin (DOX; trade name, Adriamycin) is a nonselective class I anthracycline, isolated from the pigment-producing *Streptomyces peucetius* early in the 1960s [1-3]. DOX is closely related to the natural product daunomycin (DNR), a total chemical synthesis is now possible and the structure of DOX and DNR are shown (Fig 1). DOX is one of the most-used antitumor anthracycline antibiotics that have been used for more than 40 years for the treatment of varieties of hematological malignancies and solid tumors, including leukemia, lymphoma, lung cancer, breast cancer, sarcoma, and multiple myeloma [4, 5]. The mechanisms of antitumor action of DOX remain a matter of controversy and essentially interact with the nucleus, biological membranes, and mitochondria. The following mechanisms were considered for DOX therapeutic activity: (1) intercalation into DNA, leading to inhibited synthesis of macromolecules, including DNA, RNA, and protein; (2) DNA binding, cross-linking, and alkylation; (3) interference with DNA unwinding or DNA strand separation and helicase activity; (4) initiation of DNA damage and induction of apoptosis via inhibition of topoisomerase II; (5) generation of free radicals, leading to DNA damage and/or lipid peroxidation; and (6) direct disruption of the bilayer structure in membranes [6, 7].

However, DOX has proven to be a double-edged sword because cancer patients using DOX may be complicated by acute and chronic side effects [4, 5, 8]. The acute side effects, which may develop rapidly from minutes to a week after intravenous administration of the drug, are nausea, vomiting, myelosuppression, pericarditis-myocarditis, and arrhythmias. These effects are reversible and clinically manageable. The chronic side effects, including cardiomyopathy and congestive heart failure (CHF), may develop several weeks, months, or even years after repetitive DOX administration, which are irreversible and frequently fatal, and have a grave prognosis. The cumulative dose of DOX is one of the greatest determinants of the development of CHF, and the prevalence of heart failure sharply increases at a cumulative dose of 550 mg/m^2 [3, 8]. It is noteworthy that patients treated with DOX combination with trastuzumab, taxanes, or cyclooxygenase-2 inhibitors are at greater risk of suffering cardiotoxicity along with the enhanced antitumor activity [6, 9, 10].

Others, a variety of risk factors contribute to DOX cardiotoxicity, including the rate and schedule of administration, age, gender, mediastinal radiation, history of preexisting cardiovascular disorders, hypertension, and liver disease. Among them, age seems to be the most critical risk factor since young and old patients are more prone to develop cardiomyopathy. A history of cardiovascular disease such as reduced left-ventricular ejection fraction (LVEF) and hypertension before therapy makes patients more susceptible to the cardiac toxicity of DOX [7].

The DOX cardiotoxicity has yet to find the proper prevention and treatment strategies. The objective of this chapter is to critically evaluate the latest advances regarding DOX-induced cardiomyopathy and identify primary molecular targets for new treatment. We will also explore and compare the strategies in the management of DOX cardiotoxicity to aim for a better patient care.

2. Cardiotoxicity of Doxorubicin

2.1. Morphology and Incidence of Cardiomyopathy

DOX typically induces dilated cardiomyopathy in both patients and rodents with dilation of all chambers and mural thrombi, usually observed in both ventricles [11, 12]. DOX-induced changes of microscopic features of cardiomyocytes including cytoplasmic vacuolization involving distention of sarcoplasmic reticulum and the T-tubules, myofibrillar disorganization and loss, swelling and disorganization of mitochondria and interstitial edema, increased number of lysosomes and fibroplasias, nucleus-chromatin disorganization, and replacement of chromatin by pale filaments [8, 12-14]. These changes of ultrastructural features induced by DOX characterized in patients' endomyocardial biopsies are seen also in mice, rats, and rabbits treated with adequate doses of DOX, which suggests that DOX induces morphologic damage in a species-independent pathway [15]. Most of these morphologic alternations were also replicated in vitro. DOX causes alterations in mitochondrial, nuclear, and fibrous protein structures in H9c2 myoblasts dependent on the drug concentration. Low concentrations of DOX cause mitochondrial depolarization, fragmentation, and disorganization, as well as alterations in fibrous structural proteins. More profound alterations are observed along with higher concentrations, including nuclear and mitochondrial swelling with disruption of membrane structure and extensive cytoplasm vacuolization [16]. All of these destructive actions on cardiomyocytes will eventually cause myocardial injury with significant change of the left ventricular (LV) wall thickness and increased of wall stress, which lead to the reduced ventricular ejection fraction, contractile function, diastolic dysfunction, and seriously, CHF.

DOX-induced cardiotoxicity can be divided into acute and chronic cardiotoxicity. Acute cardiotoxicity occurs rapidly, usually within a week, after initiation of a DOX regimen and the incidence is approximately 11% [11]. The manifestations are usually chest pain due to palpitations and/or myopericarditis due to premature atrial and ventricular beats, sinus tachycardia, and nonsustained ventricular tachycardia [17]. The transient electrophysiological abnormalities may present as nonspecific ST- and T-wave changes, T-wave flattening, left axis deviation, decreased QRS voltage, and prolongation of QT interval [18]. With current treatment protocols, acute cardiotoxicity is effectively managed and it is usually reversible.

Chronic cardiotoxicity is more serious and irreversible, including the development of cardiomyopathy, and ultimately CHF. It usually presents within a year of treatment and may persist or progress even after termination of treatment regimen, which may evolve into restrictive cardiomyopathy in paediatric patients and chronic dilated cardiomyopathy in adult patients [19, 20]. A number of risk factors appear to be involved in the development of clinical and subclinical cardiotoxic effects. So, patients before DOX regimen should be screened and modified risk factors to minimize the cardiotoxicity. The most significant risk factors contributing to DOX cardiotoxicity are summarized in table 1. Among them, total cumulative dose of DOX is the most critical risk factor for cardiac toxicity [21]. When the cumulative dose of the DOX exceeds 500 mg/m^2, unacceptably high incidence of DOX-induced cardiomyopathy occurs [19]. The incidence of CHF is about 4% when the dose of DOX is 500-550 mg/m^2, increases to 18% (551-600 mg/m^2), and to 36% when the dose exceeds 600 mg/m^2 [19]. After the onset of subclinical LV dysfunction, a rapid decline in LV function and heart failure occurs if DOX treatment is continued [22]. Children, adolescents and elderly patients seem to be more susceptible to the cardiac toxicity of DOX, maybe due to aging alters DO7X concentration-time course, tissue distribution, and clearance [23-28].

However, mechanisms leading to late cardiotoxicity in children differ from those causing acute cardiotoxicity in adults [29, 30]. Moreover, the incidence of cardiotoxicity was shown to higher in female patients than males for comparable doses [31, 32].

Table 1. Risk factors for Doxorubicin-induced cardiomyopathy

High total cumulative dose of DOX administered
High peak serum level of drugs
History of cardiac disease
Age, very young and very old are most susceptible
Sex
Irradiation
Combination therapy with other cardiotoxic antitumor drugs
e.g., Cyclophosphamide, taxanes (paclitaxel, docetaxel), trastuzumab, cyclooxygenase-2 inhibitor
Hypertension
Liver disease

Otherwise, late-onset chronic progressive cardiotoxicity causes LV dysfunction, arrhythmias, and CHF years to even decades after the discontinuation of chemotherapy, indicating that patients who received DOX need for a continuous follow-up of the cardiac status [33-35].

2.2. Mechanisms of Doxorubicin Cardiomyopathy

Although numerous mechanisms have been proposed to elucidate the cardiac toxicity effect of DOX, the mechanism responsible for DOX-induced cardiomyopathy remains elusive. DOX has long been said to the mechanism of cardiotoxicity different from those underlying antitumor activity, an idea which has raised hopes to design treatment protocols for protecting the heart without diminishing the drug's antitumor activity. Here, we critically describe and evaluate the latest advances that may help to shed light into the essential mechanisms of DOX-induced cardiotoxicity in experimental or clinical settings.

2.2.1. Doxorubicin-Induced Mitochondrial Dysfunction

A long list of mechanisms that have been proposed to elucidate the development of DOX-induced cardiomyopathy reveals that the cause is probably diverse and multifactorial. Increased oxidative stress due to DOX metabolism and interaction with oxygen and iron has been considered as one of the classical mechanisms of cardiotoxicity. Studies have shown that DOX, as a cationic drug, can enter and accumulate in the mitochondria, where it may inhibit the respiratory chain by interference with cardiolipin and mitochondrial DNA (mtDNA), either directly or indirectly by generating reactive oxygen species (ROS) [36-39].

DOX-induced oxidative stress can be well explained by its chemical structure. A semiquinone free radical was formed by reducing DOX, which then regenerates its parent quinone through reducing molecular oxygen to superoxide anion (O_2^-), hydrogen peroxide (H_2O_2), and hydroxyl radicals (.OH), potent members of cardiotoxic ROS (Figure 2) [40]. DOX is a favorable substrate for many oxidoreductases within cells, such as NADPH: cytochrome P450 reductase, mitochondrial NADH dehydrogenase, and xanthine oxidase [41-43]. In addition, DOX can induce transcription of endothelial nitric oxide synthase (eNOS) and increase its activity in endothelial cells [44]. And then DOX can be directly reduced by the eNOS reductase domain and enhanced the formation of superoxide [45]. Although, the Km for the reduction of DOX by eNOS is much lower than NADH dehydrogenase and cytochrome P450 reductase [45].

The principal target organelles of DOX toxicity are pointed to the mitochondria, with the significant evidence that the concentration of DOX is nearly 100-folders higher intra-mitochondrial than extracellular [36, 46, 47]. At clinical relevant plasma concentrations (0.5 – 1 μM), the intra-mitochondrial concentration of DOX should be 50 – 100 μM [48]. With the large density/volume of mitochondria in the cardiomyocytes, DOX selectively damage heart. The mitochondrial toxicity of DOX has also been observed in other tissues including lung, liver, and brain, although not as extensively as in the heart [49-52]. Mitochondria are both the important sources and targets of ROS. In mitochondria, complex I (NADH ubiquinone oxidoreductase) is considered to be the main enzyme involved in DOX redox cycling, which can reduce DOX to a highly reactive semiquinone. Compared with other tissues, such as liver, heart has much lower amount of enzymatic defenses against free radical attack [53, 54]. Actually, cardiomyocytes express low levels of catalase. When exposure to DOX, selenium-dependent GSH-peroxidase-1 is readily inactivated and cytosolic Cu-Zn superoxide dismutase decreases [53,

55, 56]. The reduction in the content/activity of antioxidant enzymes may reflect a common response to DOX treatment, at least in a specific phase [11].

DOX also binds avidly to iron, forming diverse drug-to-metal complex (1:1, 2:1, or 3:1) (Figure 1) [57]. With the presence of oxygen, DOX can directly bind iron and cycle between the iron (II) and iron (III) states, accompanied by the formation of ROS (Figure 2). Last decades, it has been reported that DOX can directly increase the labile cytosolic iron pool, which generally represents less than 5% of total cellular iron [58]. DOX and its metabolites can disrupt the Fe-S cluster of cytoplasmic aconitase and inhibit iron regulatory protein (IRP), whose function is maintaining cellular iron homeostasis [58-60]. DOX-mediated iron accumulation causing increased oxidative stress has been suggested to be a major reason for DOX cardiac toxicity and that iron chelators, such as Dexrazoxane, can effectively reduce DOX cardiotoxicity [61].

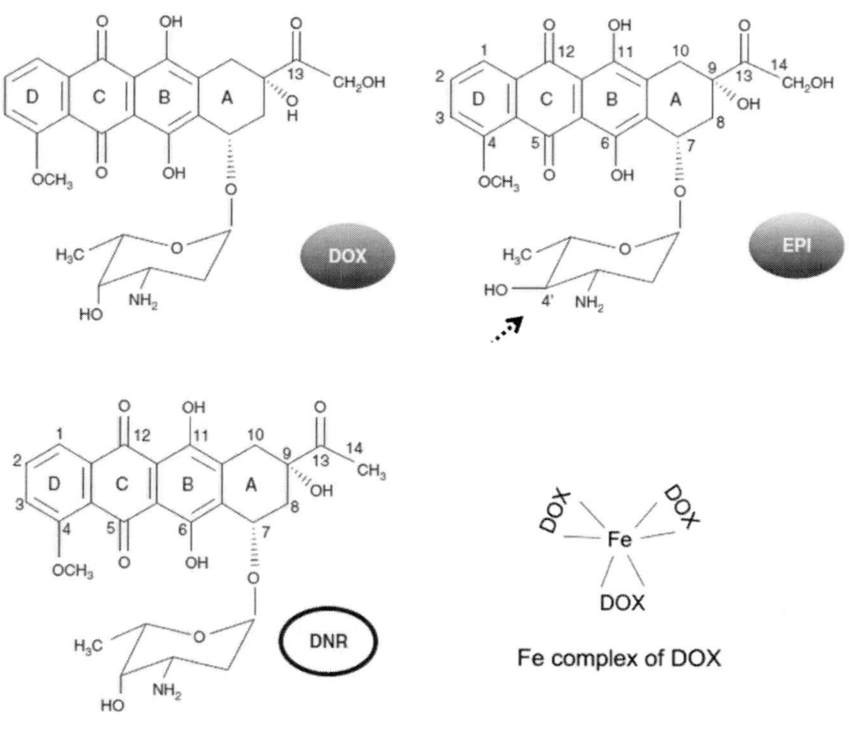

Figure 1. Structures of doxorubicin (DOX), daunorubicin (DNR), epirubicin (EPI), and the iron complex of DOX.[6, 58, 215] Dotted arrow indicates the structural modification in EPI compared with DOX (axial-to-equatorial epimerization of the hydroxyl group at C-4’ in daunosamine).

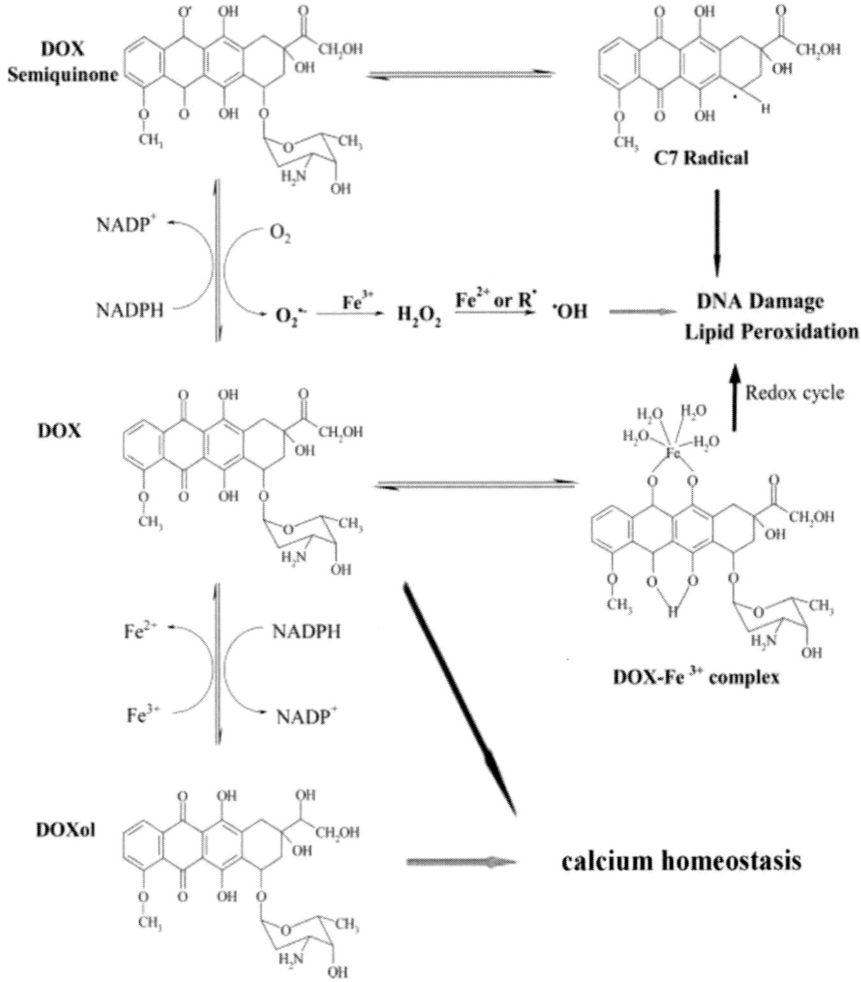

Figure 2. Illustration of DOX-mediated redox cycling and calcium homeostasis.[58, 80, 81] DOX can bind to iron forming DOX-Fe (Ⅲ) complexes, which may lead to ROS formation and cellular damage. One electron reduction of DOX generates the DOX-semiquinone that induces DNA damage and lipid peroxidation by ROS. The semiquinone radical can be transformed to a C7 radical that can also mediate cellular damage by inducing DNA damage and lipid peroxidation. The reduction of DOX by two electrons generates a secondary alcohol metabolite, doxorubicinol (DOXol). Both DOX and DOXol can interfere with the calcium homeostasis.

DOX-induced oxygen free radicals can also oxide proteins, lipids, and decrease mitochondrial membrane potential [62, 63]. ROS can damage phospholipids in membrane, increase membrane permeability, and inactivate membrane receptors and enzymes [64, 65]. DOX has a strong affinity for cardiolipin, the signature phospholipid of mitochondria, which is important for a wide variety of mitochondrial activities beyond the process of ATP production. Cardiolipin, as a cofactor for mitochondrial enzymes, is necessary for the activity of respiratory chain enzymes including cytochrome *c* oxidase and oxidoreductase [39, 66, 67]. The formation of DOX-lipid complexes leads to an inhibition of respiratory chain because cardiolipin can no longer activate enzymes [68]. With a growing body of evidences indicate that mitochondria are the preferential interacting organelles of DOX, it is not surprising that alterations of mitochondria, including stimulation of respiratory state 4 and reduction of respiratory state 3, as well as decrease the respiratory control ratio, have been observed in several different DOX models [52, 69-71].

Mitochondria are abundant in cardiac tissue and take up to 35% of the cell volume. It sustains cardiac contractile function relying upon ATP, and interference with this function is possibly leading to selective cardiotoxicity [72]. Recently, it has been suggested that DOX-induced alterations of mtDNA and interference with calcium homeostasis play an important role in mitochondrial dysfunction and subsequently onset of cardiomyopathy [14, 52, 72]. DOX reversibly intercalates with the base pairs of mtDNA, terminates the transcription and synthesis of mtDNA, and therefore interferes the synthesis of mitochondrial machinery [13, 73, 74]. The semiquinone radical may be transformed to an aglycone C7-centered radical, a potent alkylating agent, which can directly induce DNA damage (Figure 2) [47]. The alternation of mtDNA can result in respiratory chain dysfunction, which is unable to meet the high energy demands. The defective respiratory chain can subsequently generate ROS, which then in turn damage mtDNA and attack respiratory chain itself, suggesting a positive feedback loop among mtDNA damage and respiratory chain dysfunction, both progressing with time [75, 76]. It is critically important that hearts, not only from DOX-treated animals, but also from deceased patients once receiving DOX, are all observed mtDNA alterations, including rearrangements, deletions, and loss of copies [14, 77]. This strongly suggests that DOX-induced mtDNA alterations may accumulate and progress with time, during or even after treatment cessation, resulting in respiratory chain dysfunction, which, by its turn, would generate more ROS to consecutively damage mtDNA. It may explain well for the cumulative and persistent nature of the DOX cardiac toxicity.

It has been reported that mtDNA damage and the following respiratory chain deficiency precedes calcium homeostasis disruption, indicating that an early bioenergetic failure may contribute to the accumulation of calcium deposits [78]. Loss of mitochondrial calcium loading capacity is a particular aspect of DOX cardiac toxicity, which was detected in several in vivo and in vitro models [51, 52, 69, 70]. Isolated cardiac mitochondria in vivo rat studies shown that DOX inhibited the net accumulation of calcium [70, 79]. And the DOX metabolite, DOXol, has been shown to much more prone to disturb the Na+ /K+ pump of sarcolemma, the calcium pump of sarcoplasmic reticulum, and the FoF1 proton pump of mitochondria [80, 81]. While, the increased induction of the mitochondrial permeability transition (MPT) pore is the main reason for the loss of calcium loading capacity, which is a deleterious phenomenon for cells, and may result in the initiation of cell death. Oxidative stress, irreversible mitochondrial depolarization or calcium overload, leads to MPT induction and permeability of the inner mitochondrial membrane (IMM) increased [82]. MPT pore opening results in mitochondrial osmotic swelling, structural damage, and triggering the release of pro-apoptotic proteins such as cytochrome *c* or SMAC/DIABLO [83]. Several proteins have been reported to regulate the MPT, including Bcl-2 family proteins, creatine kinases (CK), hexokinase, and peripheral-type benzodiazepine receptor [84].

Loss of calcium loading capacity is considered to be an early and sensitive marker for DOX cardiotoxicity because it is observed in so many DOX cardiotoxicity models [85]. Nevertheless, there are many evidences for primary mitochondrial depolarization preceding calcium overload, and increased ROS generation [63]. It remains to be confirmed that whether the primary event is loss of calcium loading capacity or mitochondrial depolarization. Loss of calcium loading capacity has been demonstrated to be irreversible in rodent models, which again supports the cumulative and irreversible nature of DOX cardiotoxicity [70, 86, 87].

In summary, DOX interacts with oxygen and iron to increase the generation of ROS, oxidation of lipid, disruption of mtDNA, loss of calcium loading capacity, which lead to mitochondria dysfunction, and ultimately result in cardiomyopathy. Taken together, the data strongly supports that the oxidative stress is an important factor in the development of DOX cardiotoxicity. Hence, the use of antioxidants becomes a prophylactic measure to treat the cardiac deterioration. Vitamin E is one of the first antioxidants evaluated against DOX cardiotoxicity [54]. Early studies reported amelioration of DOX toxicity by vitamin E without interference with its effectiveness as chemotherapeutic agent. While other studies showed conflicting results in that vitamin E causes a potentiation of DOX toxicity or simply had no effects [54]. Further studies demonstrate that vitamin E is cardioprotective only against acute toxicity but offers no protection against the chronic cardiomyopathy of DOX [88].

Carvedilol, a clinically approved drug, is used in CHF, mild to moderate hypertension, and myocardial infarction (MI) [89]. It acts as a non-selective adrenergic blocker, and has vasodilatory properties. Besides, carvedilol has also been described to have antioxidant activity, which accounts for its additional cardio-protection [52, 85, 90, 91]. The antioxidant activity of Carvedilol is not shared by other beta-blockers, such as atenolol. Carvedilol prevents DOX-induced LV dysfunction and cardiomyocytes apoptosis, as well as H_2O_2 generation in several models [52, 85, 90]. Carvedilol also effectively attenuated cardiac mitochondrial damage in a DOX subchronic model by preventing the loss of calcium loading capacity [52, 92]. Further studies are necessary to confirm the cardioprotective action of Carvedilol does not affect the antitumor activity of DOX.

In clinical, Dexrazoxane is the only drug known to prevent DOX-induced heart injury. Dexrazoxane has two biological activities, iron chelator and topoisomerase I inhibitor. As a prodrug, it is hydrolyzed to an iron chelating agent with structural similarity to the tetra acid metal chelator EDTA, which can effectively reduce DOX cardiotoxicity and extravasation injury [93-95]. Initially, dexrazoxane (ICRF-187) was shown to protect dogs against DOX cardiotoxicity [96]. Subsequently, it was shown to exert cardioprotective effects against DOX chemotherapy in women with advanced breast cancer, without diminishing antitumor activity of DOX [97, 98]. Dexrazoxane prevents ROS-mediated initiation and perpetuation of cardiac mitochondria damage, leading to a reduced incidence of DOX-induced cardiomyopathy in animal models and humans [99]. As Dexrazoxane is a prodrug, it should be administered before DOX to get the maximal therapeutic efficacy against DOX cardiotoxicity [100].

Despite the positive impact of the antioxidants, the macromolecular damage resulting from the DOX-induced increased oxidative stress has yet to be proven to be the culprit for the cardiomyopathy, or if instead, the stress is only important in the initiation of the acute toxicity. In fact, in addition to the mixed role of antioxidants in the DOX cardiotoxicity, other potent iron chelators such as deferasirox or desferrioxamine, have failed to afford equal or better cardioprotective effect as Dexrazoxane [101, 102]. So far, it remains unclear about the mechanism of action of the iron chelators. Although the available experimental evidence strongly supports that the cardioprotective effects of Dexrazoxane is exerted by binding free iron and preventing oxidative stress on cardiac tissue, it cannot exclude that the cardioprotection of

Dexrazoxane benefits from its ability to inhibit topoisomerase II [103]. Importantly, Dexrazoxane treated patients may present lower tumor response rate and that was observed in clinical trial [104, 105]. Compared with patients receiving placebo, patients treated with Dexrazoxane had lower response rates and earlier disease progression [106].

It is also important to note that the abilities of antioxidants, iron chelators, and free redical scavengers to protect animals or patients from DOX-induced cardiomyopathy are very different. Different intracellular localization/accumulation may explain the differences in the efficacy of antioxidants or iron chelators. In fact, oxidative stress is not always an unwanted situation, which is beneficial for many normal physiological reactions. As antioxidants can neutralize ROS and decrease oxidative stress, it also can disturb the normal redox balance in cell compartments [107]. Therefore, mitochondria-directed antioxidants or iron chelators may improve their cardioprotective efficacy. Mito-Q is such an example, which prevents DOX-induced inactivation of mitochondrial complex IV [108]. Despite the promising results of many kinds of antioxidants, it remains a challenge in translation from preclinical to clinical. Numerous animal studies shown obvious protection against DOX cardiotoxicity, however, rare translates into an equal protection in humans. Different pharmacokinetics, dissimilar regulation of redox systems, or distinct cardiac metabolism may all lead to the interspecies differences.

2.2.2. Doxorubicin Activated Ubiquitin-Proteasome System

Despite the 'oxidative stress hypothesis' is widely accepted as the foremost mechanism of DOX cardiotoxicity, the use of some antioxidants has failed to date to attenuate cardiotoxicity in clinical studies. In addition, studies with potent and selective iron chelators have also yielded negative or mixed results. Therefore, alternative mechanisms have been hinted at playing important roles in DOX cardiotoxicity. Contractile dysfunction is the result of protease damage to myofibrillar proteins, which is induced by oxidative stress and elevated intracellular calcium [109, 110]. Under stress, protein folding capacity changes and the misfolded proteins accumulates within the endoplasmic reticulum (ER), a highly sensitive organelle to alterations of calcium homeostasis and free radicals [111]. Subsequently, the ubiquitin-proteasome system (UPS) is activated to remove these damaged proteins [112].

The UPS is a proteolytic system responsible for intracellular protein degradation and post-translational modifications, which consists of two main processes, ubiquitination and proteasome-mediated degradation. It is important for maintaining cellular protein functions [113-116]. Recent studies have excitingly revealed that a therapeutic dose of DOX can activate UPS-mediated proteolysis in cardiomyocytes by acting on both the ubiquitination apparatus and proteasomes [117]. The majority of studies indicated that DOX induces expression of ubiquitin E3 ligase and other proteases to promote degradation of proteins in cardiomyocytes, although a few studies showed that DOX effectively inhibits proteasome activity by forming DOX-proteasome complex [114, 118]. DOX enhances UPS-mediated degradation of essential proteins including transcription factors, survival factors (e.g., Bcl-2), and structural proteins (e.g., myofibrillar proteins) by increasing ubiquitin E3 ligase expression, which can directly cause cardiomyocyte apoptosis and impair cardiomyocyte function [110, 114, 119-121]. DOX also induces Atrogin-1, which is a muscle-specific E3 ligase promoting the degradation of muscle proteins, subsequently activates p38 MAPK pathways and causes cardiomyocyte atrophy, ventricular dilatation, and muscle wasting [122-124].

DOX can increase the amount of misfolded proteins, activate the nuclear factors of activated T-cell (NFAT) 4, and cause cardiomyocyte apoptosis by increasing ROS generation and releasing of calcium [125]. DOX causes proteasome-mediated degradation of NFAT-5, resulting in cell injury and cell death [126]. DOX can also decrease the taurine transporter (TauT) along with the reduced ability of cardiomyocytes to absorb taurine, a potent cardioprotective antioxidant amino acid [127].

Briefly, DOX-induced increasing of ubiquitin E3 ligases and other proteases result in the loss of myofibril, the impaired sarcomeric structure, the decreased of survival factors, and the increased pro-apoptotic factors. Evaluation of the protective effects of proteasome inhibitors such as bortezomib is currently ongoing in clinical studies [128].

2.2.3. Doxorubicin-Induced Alternation of Cardiac Specific Gene Expression

Available experimental evidence has indicated that DOX has diverse effects on transcription factors and expression of cardiac-specific genes encoding structural, metabolic, and enzyme protein activities. It down-regulates expression of contractile proteins, sarcoplasmic reticulum proteins, mitochondrial proteins, and others [129]. GATA-4 is a key regulator of heart development. DOX depletes GATA-4, which is known to regulate myocardial expression of sarcomeric proteins such as troponin I and myosin heavy chain [130-132]. Reduction of cardiac muscle proteins directly result in contractile dysfunction and that may be a good explanation for the loss of myofibrillar in DOX-induced cardiomyopathy. From the chronic DOX-exposed mouse, dysregulated genes are identified, including SNF1-kinase, a potential modulator of ATP levels; STARS, a hypertrophy-responsive gene; and AXUD1, a downstream target of the proapoptotic regulator AXIN1 [133]. After subchronic DOX treatment, there were significant alternations in transcription and expression of proteins in hearts, including decreased transcripts associated with fatty acid metabolism, increased expression of glycolysis genes and suppressed mitochondrial form and function related genes [86]. DOX stimulated overexpression of cardiac Adriamycin-responsive protein (CARP) in cardiomyocytes, which can suppress the transcription of cardiac troponin C and atrial natriuretic factor [134].

Moreover, acute DOX toxicity enhances the expression of several cytochrome P450 enzymes with a consequent alteration in arachidonic acid metabolism, causing progressive cardiotoxicity [135]. Chronic treatment with DOX in rats decreases organic cation/carnitine transporter (OCTN2) genes and heart fatty acid binding protein (H-FABP) in cardiac tissue and the expression of apoptotic genes p53 and CD95 are enhanced. OCTN2 and H-FABP are critical for lipid metabolism and energy generation [136].

In addition, DOX directly alters the gene expression of regulators of energy and calcium metabolism [137-140]. An animal study shown that DOX rapidly damaged or inhibited of the electron transport chain via altering transcription and translation of electron transport chain related genes, led to ATP loss and caspase 3 activation [137]. Energy production related enzymes, such as ADP/ATP translocase, phosphofructokinase, and Rieske iron-sulphur protein, are rapidly degraded as early as 2 hours after DOX administration, causing ATP depletion [139]. The expression of calcium ion homeostasis associated proteins is also altered in the hearts of rabbits chronically treated with DOX, including significantly diminished ryanodine receptors, phospholamban, calsequestrin, sarcoplasmic reticulum Ca2+-ATPase [138]. In brief, DOX-mediated suppression of mitochondrial proteins impairs energy production and its disruption of calcium ion homeostasis causes diastolic dysfunction, ultimately leading to cardiac dysfunction.

In addition to the aforementioned mechanisms, DOX-induced premature senescence in cardiomyocytes is a recently recognized novel mechanism [141]. Alterations in cardiomyocytes include structural and functional changes in mitochondria and lysosomes associated with oxidative stress [142]. And the most reliable marker of cellular senescence is the modification of the telomere-telomerase axis, together with the expression of the cell cycle inhibitors (CDKi) and p53 [142, 143]. DOX-treated neonatal cardiomyocytes showed expression of age-related proteins, including increased CDKi expression, decreased cardiac troponin I phosphorylation, decreased telomerase activity, and p53 acetylation [141].

However, it is still unknown whether the altered expression of transcription factors or specific proteins is directly mediated by ROS.

2.2.4. Doxorubicin-Induced Cardiac Inflammation

It has been proved that inflammatory cytokines are implicated in the process of several heart diseases, as a result of their negative inotropic effects and deleterious effects on LV remodeling [144, 145]. Among them, Interleukin-1 (IL-1) is closely associated with the development and progression of coronary atherosclerosis and CHF [146]. A number of studies have demonstrated that inflammation plays a role in DOX-induced cardiomyopathy. Highly upregulated expression of IL-1 in cardiomyocytes by DOX has been verified in vitro and in vivo. Recent studies have shown that DOX activates p38 MAPK and NF-κB pathways, subsequently increases the expression levels of IL-1β, IL-6, as well as tumor necrosis factor-α (TNF-α) in H9c2 cardiac cells [147]. This also has been confirmed in vivo, the expression of IL-1β is induced by DOX in a dose- and time-dependent manner associated with the severity and progress of cardiomyopathy. Systematical administration of recombinant human interleukin-1 receptor antagonist (rhIL-1Ra) has prevented the DOX cardiomyopathy [148, 149].

Interleukin-1 receptors together with Toll-like receptors (TLRs) form a receptor superfamily sharing TIR (Toll-IL-1 receptor) domains [150]. They are important components of the innate immune system and participate in the cardiac stress reaction, activating in response to pathogens and non-pathogenic components of the damaged tissue. A causal link between TLRs and the development of heart failure is indicated by a growing body of evidence from patients with heart failure and from animal models [149, 151-155]. In terms of the pathogenesis of cardiomyopathy, TLR2 and TLR4 are the most extensively studied TLRs. It has been reported that activation of NF-κB is necessary for DOX-induced cardiomyocyte apoptosis and TLR2 participates in the oxidative stress-induced activation of NF-κB in neonatal rat cardiomyocytes [156, 157]. While, the activation of NF-κB is suppressed following exposure to DOX in the TLR2-deficient mice, and there are fewer apoptotic cells than in the WT mice [153]. TLR4 activation not only results in an inflammatory response but also leads to extracellular matrix degradation, and TLR4 deficiency is able to alleviate the generation of oxidative stress, prevent GATA-4 downregulation and attenuate cardiotoxicity [152, 158]. All these provide direct evidence for a cause role of TLR-4 in cardiomyopathy.

Taken together, DOX cardiotoxicity broadly involves the activation of innate immunity and its downstream effects, although the molecular mechanism by which DOX induces cardiac inflammation has yet to be fully elucidated.

2.2.5. Doxorubicin-Induced Cardiomyocytes Loss

Cardiotoxicity is defined as a multifactorial and complex process that ultimately triggers cardiomyocyte death as the terminal event [6]. Cell death is the ultimate form of cell damage and is a direct cause of organ dysfunction. A rapidly growing body of evidence supports the concept that apoptosis and necrosis play a pivotal role in the DOX-induced cardiomyopathy and that other types of cell death, such as autophagy and senescence, are also involved in this process [159].

Under the extensively studied of the underlying mechanisms of DOX-induced cardiomyocyte apoptosis in both acute and chronic cardiotoxicity, multiple pathways are found to be involved [160-165]. Excess generation of ROS, mtDNA damage, calcium overload, generation and accumulation of ceramide, and priming of Fas are all involved in the initiation and progression of apoptosis. Calcium overload resulting from DOX treatment triggers MPT, resulting in mitochondrial membrane potential loss, mitochondrial swelling, outer-membrane permeate and rupture, cytochrome *c* and apoptosis factor release, all these lead to cell death [166, 167].

DNA lesions, p53 signal pathway and mitochondrial dysfunction also involved in DOX-induced cardiomyocyte apoptosis [84, 168, 169]. DNA damage by ROS, phosphorylation of p53 induced by DOX, and up-regulation of p53-downstream genes such as Bax, all activate the intrinsic apoptosis pathway [84]. An inhibitor of p53, Pifithrin-α attenuated the increased level of Bax and effectively inhibited DOX-induced apoptosis in vitro and in vivo [84, 169]. Mitochondrial dysfunction induced by DOX in H9c2 cardiomyoblasts was concluded to be secondary to activation of p53 [170].

The depletion of transcription factor GATA-4, which is an early event observed in the DOX cardiotoxicity, results in cardiomyocyte apoptosis [132]. GATA-4 is pivotal in heart development and it activates the antiapoptotic gene Bcl-XL to inhibit apoptotic pathway, preserving the integrity and function of mitochondria [132]. DOX also increases active GSK3β, a negative regulator of GATA-4 in the nucleus by inhibiting AKT phosphorylation [171]. Also, AKT dephosphorylation can activate caspase-3 and induce DNA damage [172].

Studies indicate that Fas-mediated apoptotic pathway is also involved in cardiomyocyte death in DOX-induced cardiomyopathy, strongly support provided by the attenuated DOX cardiotoxicity with the use of competitive inhibitor of FasL [173, 174]. In addition, TLR-2 is reported function as a novel "death receptor". There were fewer apoptotic cells in TLR-2 knockout mice than the WT mice after DOX treatment [153]. All these suggest that innate immune system is involved in the regulation of apoptotic pathway.

Necrosis is another form of cell injury, which is totally different from apoptosis and almost always detrimental. A variety of studies showed that necrosis is increased in DOX-treated animal hearts [175, 176]. Free radical scavengers protected cardiomyocytes from antracycline-induced necrosis, suggesting that oxidative stress is implicated in the cardiomyocyte necrosis [175]. The increased ROS can trigger the cell necrosis may mainly due to the mitochondrial calcium overloading, which can promote MPT pore opening and ATP depletion. If this is true, disturbance of calcium homeostasis may be a critical factor associated with the development of irreversible cardiomyopathy. Mitochondrial respiration mutilation, mtDNA damage, mitochondrial dysfunction, ATP depletion and lipid peroxidation induced by DOX all contribute to the necrosis [159, 177].

Autophagy normally occurs in the myocardium to renewal of cellular constituents. Under pathological conditions, including cardiomyopathy and heart failure, autophagy is substantially enhanced to remove protein aggregates and damaged organelles as a pro-survival pathway maintaining energy homeostasis. While, intense enhancement of autophagy can also lead to cell death [178-180].

Intracellular calcium overload not only triggers apoptosis and necrosis but also induces autophagy, which is mediated by calmodulin-dependent kinase-beta and AMP-activated protein kinase [181]. p53 and Bcl-2 family have also been shown to be involved in autophagy [181, 182]. DOX administration can enhance the autophagy and mitochondria function as the crossroads for the apoptotic, necrotic, and autophagic pathways [159, 180]. Under mild stress, autophagy functions by degrading and recycling cytoplasmic components. Apoptosis occurs because of cytochrome *c* release from mitochondria along with increasing stresses. Under extreme stress, necrosis occurs due to MPT pore opening in all mitochondria and ATP depletion. Severe stimuli can induce excessive autophagy resulting in cytosol and organelles damage, especially mitochondria and ER. In addition, excessive autophagy also induces releasing of lysosomal enzymes and cell death-inducing factors, leading to apoptosis and necrosis [183, 184]. Cell death is usually the combined result of these three types death, which converge on many levels of different pathways, such as oxidative stress, disruption of calcium homeostasis, DNA damage, mitochondria damage, and induction of proapoptotic proteins. All these events occur in DOX cardiotoxicity.

In addition to aforementioned three types of cell death, recently DOX has been also shown to induce cardiomyocyte aging. A recent study showed that exposure neonatal rat cardiomyocytes to DOX induced characteristic changes, including increased senescence-associated β-galactosidase and CDKi, decreased troponin I phosphorylation and telomerase activity, which is similar to cardiomyocytes of aged rats. Oxidative stress and p53 acetylation may be an underlying mechanism of this process [141]. Senescence mainly affects long-lived postmitotic cells, such as cardiomyocytes, and it is a risk factor for reduced cardiac function and heart diseases [185]. Oxidative stress, inflammation, reduced cellular protection and repair, altered cellular metabolism, altered protein degradation machinery and autophagy machinery, and others play vital roles in the senescence of cardiomyocytes [143]. Cardiomyocyte senescence may play a role in DOX-induced latent cardiotoxicity many years after the treatment cessation.

As mentioned above, the mechanisms of the DOX-induced cardiomyocyte death is complex and diverse. Intensive investigations on reducing DOX-induced cardiomyocyte cell death have been continuing for decades. So far, there is no drug can fully and effectively block cardiomyocyte death. Although, mitochondria seems the initiators or at least magnifiers of cell death, targeting the mitochondrial dysfunction to prevent cell death may prove of limited value, because apoptotic signaling originating from other organelles was also important in the context of DOX cardiotoxicity [186]. Sarcoplasmic reticulum is one of those organelles, activating caspase-12 after DOX treatment, ultimately leading to apoptosis [187].

3. Strategies to Reduce the Doxorubicin-Induced Cardiotoxicity

3.1. Prevention

In clinical, the first line of defense against DOX cardiotoxicity is limiting the cumulative dose of DOX. To minimize the cumulative dose of DOX, one strategy is combined chemotherapy, for example, DOX combined with cyclophosphamide (CTX). Apart from the total amount of DOX limitation, many attempts have been made to develop additional strategies to prevent DOX-induced cardiomyopathy without attenuating its antitumor effect. Alternative drug-delivery methods, DOX analogues, antioxidants, iron chelators and protease inhibitors have all been tested in rodents or in humans (Table 2).

Table 2. Potential strategies to reduce Doxorubicin-induced cardiomyopathy

Limiting the cumulative dose of DOX
Alternative methods for drug delivery
Continuous slow infusion
Liposome-encapsulated DOX (Caelyx (Doxil in USA), Myocet)
Nanoparticle
DOX analogues
EPI
Antioxidants, free radical scavengers and iron-chelating agents
Probucol
Dexrazoxane (only cardioprotective drug currently available clinically)
Carvedilol (clinically approved drug)
Melatonin
Frederine
Mito-Q
Inhibition of increased [Ca^{2+}]
Carnitine
Proteasome inhibitors
Bortezomib

3.1.1. Alternative Methods for Drug Delivery

Slow Infusion

The clinical standard procedure for DOX administration is rapid intravenous infusion over 15 to 20 minutes. Clinical studies comparing the cardiotoxicity and antitumor activity of this rapid infusion with continuous infusion over a 6-hours period or over a period of 48 to 96 hours have revealed that the slower infusion significantly reduces the severe morphologic changes in the endomyocardial biopsies and the incidence of CHF, without diminishing its antitumor activity in patients [188-190]. The safety and efficacy of slow infusion in adult patients have been confirmed ever since, however, it remains controversial when this schedule is adopted in pediatric settings. A study showed that children treated with DOX over 24 hours (60 mg/m^2) or over 72 hours (75 mg/m^2) had lower incidence of CHF than the historical control patients with bolus infusion [191]. In contrast, in a trial of children with acute lymphoblastic leukemia who were randomized to receive continuous infusion over 48 hours or bolus infusion within 1 hour of DOX, there was no advantage of avoiding cardiomyopathy or inadequate LV hypertrophy [192]. Since not all of the patients benefit of slow infusion, other better cardioprotective strategies should be explored.

Liposomal Formulations

Long term exposure to drugs at moderate concentrations is generally believed to be safer than a pulsed supply of the drug at higher concentrations. Drug carriers that assist preferential distribution of DOX to tumors while not exposing cardiac tissue potentially improve the efficacy and/or cardiac safety. A tumor-targeted and/or sustained-release drug delivery system such as liposomes and nanoparticles is a promising approach to increase the efficacy and reduce the side effects of DOX.

In terms of efficacy and cardiactoxicity, liposome-encapsulated DOX formulations have been assessed and shown to be superior to conventional DOX in the clinical setting [193-196]. Two liposome formulations have been approved for clinical use by the US Food and Drug Administration. They are Caelyx (Doxil in USA), a sterically stabilized DOX polyethylenglycol-coated formulation; and Myocet, a non-pegylated liposome-encapsulated DOX formulation.

Initially, liposomal drug delivery system has shown great promise. Yet, it has also been demonstrated some critical shortcomings, including leakage, easy recognition, and removal due to the particles' composition and size [197, 198]. In order to prevent initial drug leakage and prolong circulation time, the liposomes were coated with polyethylene glycol (PEG). Pegylation allows the liposomes to circulate in the blood longer, and the "stealth" properties permit it undetected by the mononuclear phagocyte system [199].

The pegylated liposomal-DOX (PLD) causes less alopecia, vomiting, nausea, stomatitis, myelosuppression, and cardiotoxicity than the conventional DOX [193, 194, 200, 201]. The reduced cardiotoxicity of PLD was also confirmed in other trials evaluating the PLD-docetaxel combination in the first-line therapy of the metastatic breast cancer [202-204]. However, hand and foot syndrome (palmar-plantar erythrodysesthesia syndrome, PPE) is a frequent adverse effect of PLD. The incidence of this syndrome is dependent on the dose and the administration interval, so the primarily strategy to manage it is dose reduction and cycle duration prolongation [205]. It's conceivable that docetaxel, especially paclitaxel, can interfere with the pharmacokinetics of PLD, with the slowed clearance of PLD, and thereby enhance the incidence of skin toxicity [206].

The change of the pharmacokinetic parameters of the non-pegylated liposomal-DOX formulation is less significant than that of PLD, but still more favorable than the free DOX, especially in the treatment of metastatic breast cancer. Non-pegylated liposomal-DOX achieves the same objective response as the conventional DOX, but with infrequent cardiotoxicity and PPE [196]. In a randomized phase III study of metastatic breast cancer patients, the non-pegylated liposomal-DOX plus CTX achieved the same objective response rates as the conventional DOX plus CTX but lower cardiotoxicity. The median cumulative dose of DOX at the onset of cardiotoxicity in the liposomal DOX/CTX (2220 mg/m^2) was more than in the free DOX/CTX (480 mg/m^2) [207].

Nanoparticles

As discussed above, the development of new drug delivery systems to improve the efficiency of drug delivery as well as reduce the side effects is continuously being explored. Formerly, macromolecular materials have been used successfully as potential delivery carriers, such as polyethyleneimine (PEI) and dextran [208]. Recently, a study demonstrated dextran-graft-PEI nanoparticles loaded with DOX has higher cytotoxicity than free DOX in SaOS-2 and MG-63 cells [209]. Specific delivery to tumors is another characteristic of DOX-coupled nanoparticles. For this reason, DOX-loaded dextran-PEI nanoparticles increase the margin of safety in combination with fewer side effects. As a drug delivery system, another advantage of nanoparticles is that they can be easily manufactured, with the added benefits of low toxicity and biodegradability. The combination delivery systems are now commonly used to effectively treat cancer.

Another recent study about novel formulation of DOX is encapsulation DOX into chitosan-based drug delivery system via the complex coacervation method with dextran sulfate [210]. The DOX nanoparticles reduced tumor growth, metastasis to the lungs and tumor-associated osteolysis in orthotopic osteosarcoma bearing mice. It is important that the nanoparticles did not cause side effects in mice, specifically to the heart or skin. Thus, DOX-containing nanoparticles may prove to be useful clinically. However, further studies are necessary to verify such formulations in clinically relevant animal tumor models.

3.1.2. Analogs

Last 3 decades have witnessed attempts to improve the therapeutic and pharmacological properties of the natural compounds via modifications in the basic structure of anthracyclines. This has resulted in about 2000 analogs, though only few analogs have reached the stage of clinical development and approval. Among them, epirubicin (EPI), which derived from a semisynthetic derivative of DOX by an axial-to-equatorial epimerization of the hydroxyl group at C-4' in daunosamine, enjoy large popularity as useful alternative to DOX (Figure 1). This modification has little effect on the mechanism and spectrum of antitumor activity compared to DOX, however, leads to pharmacokinetic and metabolic changes. Due to the different pharmacokinetic and metabolic properties, duplication of cumulative doses of EPI compared to DOX has at least equal efficacy without increasing cardiotoxicity [211, 212]. The median dose to develop cardiotoxicity is 935 mg/m^2 (EPI) compared to 468 mg/m^2 (DOX). The median cumulative dose of EPI associated with development of symptomatic CHF is 1,134 mg/m^2 compared to 492 mg/m^2 (DOX) [213]. Directly comparing EPI and DOX head-to-head in metastatic breast cancer and also in the adjuvant setting, showed that CTX combination with DOX was inferior to combination with EPI in relapse-free survival (RFS) [214]. Khasraw et al. summarized the published clinical trials investigating EPI in the treatment of early and advanced breast cancer, and showed that at equimolar doses, the efficacy of EPI is similar to DOX while EPI has more favorable hematologic and non-hematologic toxicity, particularly cardiotoxicity [215]. However, as with DOX, the cardiotoxicity of EPI is dependent on the cumulative dose, and 900 mg/m^2 was cautiously recommended as the maximum cumulative dose of EPI [216]. Thus, EPI alternative to DOX, does not eliminate the risk of developing chronic cardiotoxicity. Therefore, there is urgent need to develop new and better analogues with the properties of lower cardiotoxicity and higher antitumor activity.

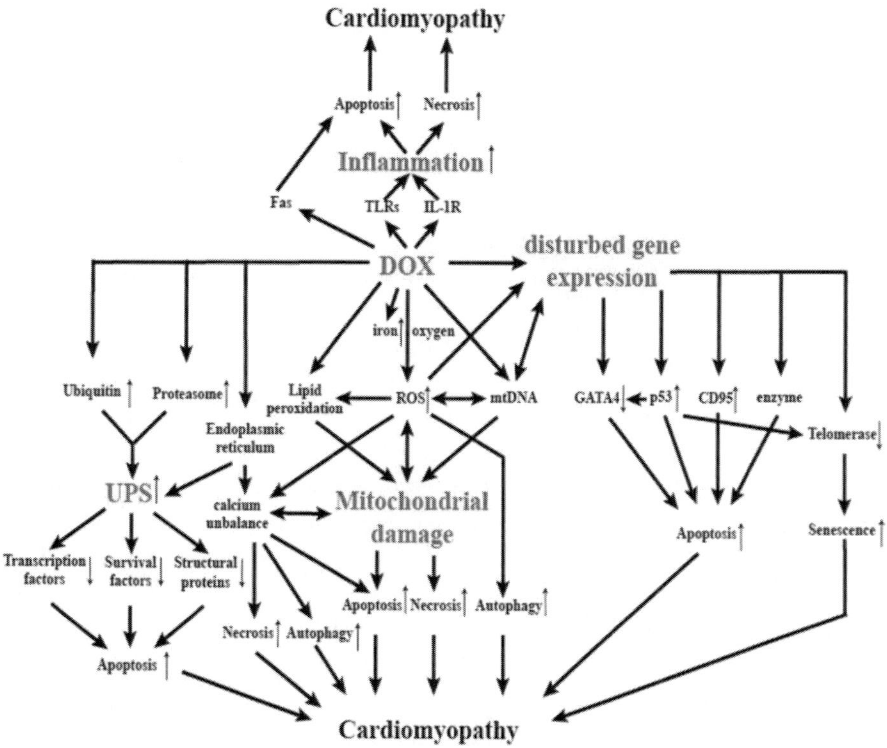

Figure 3. A summary of potential mechanisms involved in DOX-induced cardiomyopathy as described in the text. The major mechanism involves mitochondrial dysfunction induced by increased ROS, lipid peroxidation, mtDNA damage, and overloading calcium. Meanwhile, DOX activates ubiquitin-proteasome system (UPS) causing the balance of the protein system to shift toward proapoptosis, down regulation survival factors, degradation of structural proteins such as myofilament proteins. DOX also activates innate immunity and promotes inflammation. In addition, DOX disturbes gene expression resulting in reduced cardiac-specific gene expression, triggers apoptosis, and induces cardiac premature senescence. All these events subsequently induce cardiomyocytes death by apoptosis, necrosis, and autophagy or cell senescence, which ultimately causes cardiomyopathy.

3.2. Treatment

Currently, there is no specific and effective therapy for DOX-induced cardiomyopathy. In the case of established CHF, there are only some strategies to relieve symptoms and improve the functional status of the patients, including low salt diet, diuretics, β-blockers, as well as angiotensin converting enzyme inhibitors. For patients with end-stage CHF, cardiac transplantation remains an important option.

Conclusion

Doxorubicin is one of the most effective and widely used antitumor agents, but its dose-dependent and cumulative cardiotoxicity leads to substantial morbidity and mortality for cancer survivors. DOX cardiotoxicity remains a huge challenge in oncology. Despite intensive efforts, the underlying mechanisms of DOX cardiotoxicity remain to be poorly understood and consequently the means available for clinicians to prevent or effectively manage DOX cardiotoxicity are very limited. There is no single drug that is able to completely prevent DOX cardiotoxicity. The preclinically potent cardioprotective agents fail to provide the expected protection in humans may be well elucidated by the multifactorial nature of the DOX effects and the domino effect that each molecular event may trigger (Figure 3).

To understand the essential mechanisms responsible for DOX cardiotoxicity, much is yet to be done and further studies will continuously be conducted. There is a growing demand for preventive strategies and effective therapies against DOX cardiotoxicity, particularly late-onset cardiomyopathy to prevent DOX-induced premature cardiomyocyte death in cancer patients.

References

[1] Arcamone, F; Cassinelli, G; Fantini, G; Grein, A; Orezzi, P; Pol, C, et al. Adriamycin, 14-hydroxydaunomycin, a new antitumor antibiotic from S. peucetius var. caesius. *Biotechnology and bioengineering,* 1969, 11, 1101-10.

[2] Di Marco, A; Gaetani, M; Scarpinato, B. Adriamycin (NSC-123, 127): a new antibiotic with antitumor activity. *Cancer chemotherapy reports* Part 1, 1969, 53, 33-7.

[3] Bonadonna, G; Monfardini, S; De Lena, M; Fossati-Bellani, F; Beretta, G. Phase I and preliminary phase II evaluation of adriamycin (NSC 123127). *Cancer research,* 1970, 30, 2572-82.

[4] Carvalho, C; Santos, RX; Cardoso, S; Correia, S; Oliveira, PJ; Santos, MS, et al. Doxorubicin: the good, the bad and the ugly effect. *Current medicinal chemistry*, 2009, 16, 3267-85.

[5] Tacar, O; Sriamornsak, P; Dass, CR. Doxorubicin: an update on anticancer molecular action, toxicity and novel drug delivery systems. *The Journal of pharmacy and pharmacology*, 2013, 65, 157-70.

[6] Minotti, G; Menna, P; Salvatorelli, E; Cairo, G; Gianni, L. Anthracyclines: molecular advances and pharmacologic developments in antitumor activity and cardiotoxicity. *Pharmacological reviews,* 2004, 56, 185-229.

[7] Carvalho, FS; Burgeiro, A; Garcia, R; Moreno, AJ; Carvalho, RA; Oliveira, PJ. Doxorubicin-Induced Cardiotoxicity: From Bioenergetic Failure and Cell Death to Cardiomyopathy. *Medicinal research reviews,* 2013.

[8] Chatterjee, K; Zhang, J; Honbo, N; Karliner, JS. Doxorubicin cardiomyopathy. *Cardiology,* 2010, 115, 155-62.

[9] Tan-Chiu, E; Yothers, G; Romond, E; Geyer, CE, Jr.; Ewer, M; Keefe, D, et al. Assessment of cardiac dysfunction in a randomized trial comparing doxorubicin and cyclophosphamide followed by paclitaxel, with or without trastuzumab as adjuvant therapy in node-positive, human epidermal growth factor receptor 2-overexpressing breast cancer: NSABP B-31. Journal of clinical oncology : official journal of the *American Society of Clinical Oncology,* 2005, 23, 7811-9.

[10] Gianni, L; Salvatorelli, E; Minotti, G. Anthracycline cardiotoxicity in breast cancer patients: synergism with trastuzumab and taxanes. *Cardiovascular toxicology*, 2007, 7, 67-71.

[11] Takemura, G; Fujiwara, H. Doxorubicin-induced cardiomyopathy from the cardiotoxic mechanisms to management. *Progress in cardiovascular diseases,* 2007, 49, 330-52.

[12] Billingham, ME; Mason, JW; Bristow, MR; Daniels, JR. Anthracycline cardiomyopathy monitored by morphologic changes. Cancer treatment reports, 1978, 62, 865-72.

[13] Unverferth, DV; Magorien, RD; Unverferth, BP; Talley, RL; Balcerzak, SP; Baba, N. Human myocardial morphologic and functional changes in the first 24 hours after doxorubicin administration. *Cancer treatment reports,* 1981, 65, 1093-7.

[14] Lebrecht, D; Kokkori, A; Ketelsen, UP; Setzer, B; Walker, UA. Tissue-specific mtDNA lesions and radical-associated mitochondrial

dysfunction in human hearts exposed to doxorubicin. *The Journal of pathology,* 2005, 207, 436-44.

[15] Singal, PK; Li, T; Kumar, D; Danelisen, I; Iliskovic, N. Adriamycin-induced heart failure: mechanism and modulation. *Molecular and cellular biochemistry,* 2000, 207, 77-86.

[16] Sardao, VA; Oliveira, PJ; Holy, J; Oliveira, CR; Wallace, KB. Morphological alterations induced by doxorubicin on H9c2 myoblasts: nuclear, mitochondrial, and cytoskeletal targets. *Cell biology and toxicology,* 2009, 25, 227-43.

[17] Steinberg, JS; Cohen, AJ; Wasserman, AG; Cohen, P; Ross, AM. Acute arrhythmogenicity of doxorubicin administration. *Cancer,* 1987, 60, 1213-8.

[18] Singal, PK; Iliskovic, N. Doxorubicin-induced cardiomyopathy. *The New England journal of medicine,* 1998, 339, 900-5.

[19] Lefrak, EA; Pitha, J; Rosenheim, S; Gottlieb, JA. A clinicopathologic analysis of adriamycin cardiotoxicity. *Cancer,* 1973, 32, 302-14.

[20] Praga, C; Beretta, G; Vigo, PL; Lenaz, GR; Pollini, C; Bonadonna, G, et al. Adriamycin cardiotoxicity: a survey of 1273 patients. *Cancer treatment reports,* 1979, 63, 827-34.

[21] Von Hoff, DD; Layard, MW; Basa, P; Davis, HL, Jr.; Von Hoff, AL; Rozencweig, M, et al. Risk factors for doxorubicin-induced congestive heart failure. *Annals of internal medicine,* 1979, 91, 710-7.

[22] Jain, D. Cardiotoxicity of doxorubicin and other anthracycline derivatives. Journal of nuclear cardiology : official publication of the *American Society of Nuclear Cardiology,* 2000, 7, 53-62.

[23] Lipshultz, SE. Exposure to anthracyclines during childhood causes cardiac injury. *Seminars in oncology,* 2006, 33, S8-14.

[24] Kremer, LC; van Dalen, EC; Offringa, M; Voute, PA. Frequency and risk factors of anthracycline-induced clinical heart failure in children: a systematic review. *Annals of oncology : official journal of the European Society for Medical Oncology* / ESMO, 2002, 13, 503-12.

[25] Doyle, JJ; Neugut, AI; Jacobson, JS; Grann, VR; Hershman, DL. Chemotherapy and cardiotoxicity in older breast cancer patients: a population-based study. Journal of clinical oncology : official journal of *the American Society of Clinical Oncology,* 2005, 23, 8597-605.

[26] Cusack, BJ; Musser, B; Gambliel, H; Hadjokas, NE; Olson, RD. Effect of dexrazoxane on doxorubicin pharmacokinetics in young and old rats. *Cancer chemotherapy and pharmacology*, 2003, 51, 139-46.

[27] Robert, J; Hoerni, B. Age dependence of the early-phase pharmacokinetics of doxorubicin. *Cancer research,* 1983, 43, 4467-9.

[28] Li, J; Gwilt, PR. The effect of age on the early disposition of doxorubicin. *Cancer chemotherapy and pharmacology,* 2003, 51, 395-402.

[29] De Angelis, A; Piegari, E; Cappetta, D; Marino, L; Filippelli, A; Berrino, L, et al. Anthracycline cardiomyopathy is mediated by depletion of the cardiac stem cell pool and is rescued by restoration of progenitor cell function. *Circulation,* 2010, 121, 276-92.

[30] Lipshultz, SE; Rifai, N; Dalton, VM; Levy, DE; Silverman, LB; Lipsitz, SR, et al. The effect of dexrazoxane on myocardial injury in doxorubicin-treated children with acute lymphoblastic leukemia. *The New England journal of medicine,* 2004, 351, 145-53.

[31] Lipshultz, SE; Lipsitz, SR; Mone, SM; Goorin, AM; Sallan, SE; Sanders, SP, et al. Female sex and drug dose as risk factors for late cardiotoxic effects of doxorubicin therapy for childhood cancer. *The New England journal of medicine,* 1995, 332, 1738-43.

[32] Silber, JH; Jakacki, RI; Larsen, RL; Goldwein, JW; Barber, G. Increased risk of cardiac dysfunction after anthracyclines in girls. *Medical and pediatric oncology,* 1993, 21, 477-9.

[33] Haq, MM; Legha, SS; Choksi, J; Hortobagyi, GN; Benjamin, RS; Ewer, M, et al. Doxorubicin-induced congestive heart failure in adults. *Cancer,* 1985, 56, 1361-5.

[34] Schwartz, RG; McKenzie, WB; Alexander, J; Sager, P; D'Souza, A; Manatunga, A, et al. Congestive heart failure and left ventricular dysfunction complicating doxorubicin therapy. Seven-year experience using serial radionuclide angiocardiography. *The American journal of medicine*, 1987, 82, 1109-18.

[35] Lipshultz, SE; Colan, SD; Gelber, RD; Perez-Atayde, AR; Sallan, SE; Sanders, SP. Late cardiac effects of doxorubicin therapy for acute lymphoblastic leukemia in childhood. *The New England journal of medicine,* 1991, 324, 808-15.

[36] Sarvazyan, N. Visualization of doxorubicin-induced oxidative stress in isolated cardiac myocytes. *The American journal of physiology,* 1996, 271, H2079-85.

[37] Zhou, S; Palmeira, CM; Wallace, KB. Doxorubicin-induced persistent oxidative stress to cardiac myocytes. *Toxicology letters,* 2001, 121, 151-7.

[38] Adachi, K; Fujiura, Y; Mayumi, F; Nozuhara, A; Sugiu, Y; Sakanashi, T, et al. A deletion of mitochondrial DNA in murine doxorubicin-induced cardiotoxicity. *Biochemical and biophysical research communications,* 1993, 195, 945-51.

[39] Goormaghtigh, E; Huart, P; Praet, M; Brasseur, R; Ruysschaert, JM. Structure of the adriamycin-cardiolipin complex. Role in mitochondrial toxicity. *Biophysical chemistry,* 1990, 35, 247-57.

[40] Menna, P; Salvatorelli, E; Minotti, G. Cardiotoxicity of antitumor drugs. *Chemical research in toxicology,* 2008, 21, 978-89.

[41] Doroshow, JH. Anthracycline antibiotic-stimulated superoxide, hydrogen peroxide, and hydroxyl radical production by NADH dehydrogenase. *Cancer research,* 1983, 43, 4543-51.

[42] Doroshow, JH; Davies, KJ. Redox cycling of anthracyclines by cardiac mitochondria. II. Formation of superoxide anion, hydrogen peroxide, and hydroxyl radical. *The Journal of biological chemistry,* 1986, 261, 3068-74.

[43] Doroshow, JH. Effect of anthracycline antibiotics on oxygen radical formation in rat heart. *Cancer research,* 1983, 43, 460-72.

[44] Vasquez-Vivar, J; Martasek, P; Hogg, N; Masters, BS; Pritchard, KA, Jr.; Kalyanaraman, B. Endothelial nitric oxide synthase-dependent superoxide generation from adriamycin. *Biochemistry,* 1997, 36, 11293-7.

[45] Kalivendi, SV; Kotamraju, S; Zhao, H; Joseph, J; Kalyanaraman, B. Doxorubicin-induced apoptosis is associated with increased transcription of endothelial nitric-oxide synthase. Effect of antiapoptotic antioxidants and calcium. *The Journal of biological chemistry,* 2001, 276, 47266-76.

[46] Konorev, EA; Kennedy, MC; Kalyanaraman, B. Cell-permeable superoxide dismutase and glutathione peroxidase mimetics afford superior protection against doxorubicin-induced cardiotoxicity: the role of reactive oxygen and nitrogen intermediates. *Archives of biochemistry and biophysics,* 1999, 368, 421-8.

[47] Jung, K; Reszka, R. Mitochondria as subcellular targets for clinically useful anthracyclines. *Advanced drug delivery reviews,* 2001, 49, 87-105.

[48] Davies, KJ; Doroshow, JH. Redox cycling of anthracyclines by cardiac mitochondria. I. Anthracycline radical formation by NADH dehydrogenase. *The Journal of biological chemistry,* 1986, 261, 3060-7.

[49] Cardoso, S; Santos, RX; Carvalho, C; Correia, S; Pereira, GC; Pereira, SS, et al. Doxorubicin increases the susceptibility of brain mitochondria to Ca(2+)-induced permeability transition and oxidative damage. *Free radical biology & medicine,* 2008, 45, 1395-402.

[50] Machado, NG; Baldeiras, I; Pereira, GC; Pereira, SP; Oliveira, PJ. Sub-chronic administration of doxorubicin to Wistar rats results in oxidative stress and unaltered apoptotic signaling in the lung. *Chemico-biological interactions,* 2010, 188, 478-86.

[51] Ascensao, A; Lumini-Oliveira, J; Machado, NG; Ferreira, RM; Goncalves, IO; Moreira, AC, et al. Acute exercise protects against calcium-induced cardiac mitochondrial permeability transition pore opening in doxorubicin-treated rats. *Clinical science,* 2011, 120, 37-49.

[52] Santos, DL; Moreno, AJ; Leino, RL; Froberg, MK; Wallace, KB. Carvedilol protects against doxorubicin-induced mitochondrial cardiomyopathy. *Toxicology and applied pharmacology*, 2002, 185, 218-27.

[53] Doroshow, JH; Locker, GY; Myers, CE. Enzymatic defenses of the mouse heart against reactive oxygen metabolites: alterations produced by doxorubicin. *The Journal of clinical investigation,* 1980, 65, 128-35.

[54] Quiles, JL; Huertas, JR; Battino, M; Mataix, J; Ramirez-Tortosa, MC. Antioxidant nutrients and adriamycin toxicity. *Toxicology,* 2002, 180, 79-95.

[55] Li, T; Danelisen, I; Singal, PK. Early changes in myocardial antioxidant enzymes in rats treated with adriamycin. *Molecular and cellular biochemistry, 2002*, 232, 19-26.

[56] Sazuka, Y; Tanizawa, H; Takino, Y. Effect of adriamycin on the activities of superoxide dismutase, glutathione peroxidase and catalase in tissues of mice. Japanese journal of cancer research : *Gann,* 1989, 80, 89-94.

[57] Myers, C; Gianni, L; Zweier, J; Muindi, J; Sinha, BK; Eliot, H. Role of iron in adriamycin biochemistry. *Federation proceedings,* 1986, 45, 2792-7.

[58] Xu, X; Persson, HL; Richardson, DR. Molecular pharmacology of the interaction of anthracyclines with iron. *Molecular pharmacology,* 2005, 68, 261-71.

[59] Cairo, G; Recalcati, S. Iron-regulatory proteins: molecular biology and pathophysiological implications. *Expert reviews in molecular medicine,* 2007, 9, 1-13.

[60] Minotti, G; Ronchi, R; Salvatorelli, E; Menna, P; Cairo, G. Doxorubicin irreversibly inactivates iron regulatory proteins 1 and 2 in cardiomyocytes: evidence for distinct metabolic pathways and implications for iron-mediated cardiotoxicity of antitumor therapy. *Cancer research,* 2001, 61, 8422-8.

[61] Ducroq, J; Moha ou Maati, H; Guilbot, S; Dilly, S; Laemmel, E; Pons-Himbert, C, et al. Dexrazoxane protects the heart from acute doxorubicin-induced QT prolongation: a key role for I(Ks). *British journal of pharmacology,* 2010, 159, 93-101.

[62] Berthiaume, JM; Wallace, KB. Adriamycin-induced oxidative mitochondrial cardiotoxicity. *Cell biology and toxicology,* 2007, 23, 15-25.

[63] Kuznetsov, AV; Margreiter, R; Amberger, A; Saks, V; Grimm, M. Changes in mitochondrial redox state, membrane potential and calcium precede mitochondrial dysfunction in doxorubicin-induced cell death. *Biochimica et biophysica acta,* 2011, 1813, 1144-52.

[64] Marcillat, O; Zhang, Y; Davies, KJ. Oxidative and non-oxidative mechanisms in the inactivation of cardiac mitochondrial electron transport chain components by doxorubicin. *The Biochemical journal,* 1989, 259, 181-9.

[65] Yoon, SB; Kajiyama, K; Hino, Y; Sugiyama, M; Ogura, R. Effect of adriamycin on lipid peroxide, glutathione peroxidase and respiratory responses of mitochondria from the heart, liver and kidney. *The Kurume medical journal,* 1983, 30, 1-4.

[66] Parker, MA; King, V; Howard, KP. Nuclear magnetic resonance study of doxorubicin binding to cardiolipin containing magnetically oriented phospholipid bilayers. *Biochimica et biophysica acta,* 2001, 1514, 206-16.

[67] Claypool, SM; Koehler, CM. The complexity of cardiolipin in health and disease. *Trends in biochemical sciences,* 2012, 37, 32-41.

[68] Goormaghtigh, E; Huart, P; Brasseur, R; Ruysschaert, JM. Mechanism of inhibition of mitochondrial enzymatic complex I-III by adriamycin derivatives. *Biochimica et biophysica acta,* 1986, 861, 83-94.

[69] Oliveira, PJ; Wallace, KB. Depletion of adenine nucleotide translocator protein in heart mitochondria from doxorubicin-treated rats--relevance for mitochondrial dysfunction. *Toxicology,* 2006, 220, 160-8.

[70] Zhou, S; Starkov, A; Froberg, MK; Leino, RL; Wallace, KB. Cumulative and irreversible cardiac mitochondrial dysfunction induced by doxorubicin. *Cancer research,* 2001, 61, 771-7.

[71] Pereira, GC; Pereira, SP; Pereira, CV; Lumini, JA; Magalhaes, J; Ascensao, A, et al. Mitochondrionopathy phenotype in doxorubicin-treated Wistar rats depends on treatment protocol and is cardiac-specific. *PloS one,* 2012, 7, e38867.

[72] Wallace, KB. Adriamycin-induced interference with cardiac mitochondrial calcium homeostasis. *Cardiovascular toxicology,* 2007, 7, 101-7.

[73] Ashley, N; Poulton, J. Mitochondrial DNA is a direct target of anti-cancer anthracycline drugs. *Biochemical and biophysical research communications,* 2009, 378, 450-5.

[74] Ellis, CN; Ellis, MB; Blakemore, WS. Effect of adriamycin on heart mitochondrial DNA. *The Biochemical journal,* 1987, 245, 309-12.

[75] Serrano, J; Palmeira, CM; Kuehl, DW; Wallace, KB. Cardioselective and cumulative oxidation of mitochondrial DNA following subchronic doxorubicin administration. *Biochimica et biophysica acta,* 1999, 1411, 201-5.

[76] Palmeira, CM; Serrano, J; Kuehl, DW; Wallace, KB. Preferential oxidation of cardiac mitochondrial DNA following acute intoxication with doxorubicin. *Biochimica et biophysica acta,* 1997, 1321, 101-6.

[77] Lebrecht, D; Setzer, B; Ketelsen, UP; Haberstroh, J; Walker, UA. Time-dependent and tissue-specific accumulation of mtDNA and respiratory chain defects in chronic doxorubicin cardiomyopathy. *Circulation,* 2003, 108, 2423-9.

[78] Lebrecht, D; Kirschner, J; Geist, A; Haberstroh, J; Walker, UA. Respiratory chain deficiency precedes the disrupted calcium homeostasis in chronic doxorubicin cardiomyopathy. Cardiovascular pathology : the official journal of the Society for Cardiovascular *Pathology,* 2010, 19, e167-74.

[79] Solem, LE; Henry, TR; Wallace, KB. Disruption of mitochondrial calcium homeostasis following chronic doxorubicin administration. *Toxicology and applied pharmacology*, 1994, 129, 214-22.

[80] Olson, RD; Mushlin, PS; Brenner, DE; Fleischer, S; Cusack, BJ; Chang, BK, et al. Doxorubicin cardiotoxicity may be caused by its metabolite, doxorubicinol. *Proceedings of the National Academy of Sciences of the United States of America*, 1988, 85, 3585-9.

[81] Mordente, A; Meucci, E; Silvestrini, A; Martorana, GE; Giardina, B. New developments in anthracycline-induced cardiotoxicity. *Current medicinal chemistry,* 2009, 16, 1656-72.

[82] Rasola, A; Bernardi, P. Mitochondrial permeability transition in Ca(2+)-dependent apoptosis and necrosis. *Cell calcium,* 2011, 50, 222-33.

[83] Baines, CP. The molecular composition of the mitochondrial permeability transition pore. *Journal of molecular and cellular cardiology,* 2009, 46, 850-7.

[84] Liu, J; Mao, W; Ding, B; Liang, CS. ERKs/p53 signal transduction pathway is involved in doxorubicin-induced apoptosis in H9c2 cells and cardiomyocytes. *American journal of physiology Heart and circulatory physiology, 2008*, 295, H1956-65.

[85] Oliveira, PJ; Bjork, JA; Santos, MS; Leino, RL; Froberg, MK; Moreno, AJ, et al. Carvedilol-mediated antioxidant protection against doxorubicin-induced cardiac mitochondrial toxicity. *Toxicology and applied pharmacology,* 2004, 200, 159-68.

[86] Berthiaume, JM; Wallace, KB. Persistent alterations to the gene expression profile of the heart subsequent to chronic Doxorubicin treatment. *Cardiovascular toxicology, 2007*, 7, 178-91.

[87] Richard, C; Ghibu, S; Delemasure-Chalumeau, S; Guilland, JC; Des Rosiers, C; Zeller, M, et al. Oxidative stress and myocardial gene alterations associated with Doxorubicin-induced cardiotoxicity in rats persist for 2 months after treatment cessation. *The Journal of pharmacology and experimental therapeutics,* 2011, 339, 807-14.

[88] Hermansen, K; Wassermann, K. The effect of vitamin E and selenium on doxorubicin (Adriamycin) induced delayed toxicity in mice. *Acta pharmacologica et toxicologica,* 1986, 58, 31-7.

[89] Dunn, CJ; Lea, AP; Wagstaff, AJ. Carvedilol. A reappraisal of its pharmacological properties and therapeutic use in cardiovascular disorders. *Drugs,* 1997, 54, 161-85.

[90] Spallarossa, P; Garibaldi, S; Altieri, P; Fabbi, P; Manca, V; Nasti, S, et al. Carvedilol prevents doxorubicin-induced free radical release and apoptosis in cardiomyocytes in vitro. *Journal of molecular and cellular cardiology,* 2004, 37, 837-46.

[91] Machado, V; Cabral, A; Monteiro, P; Goncalves, L; Providencia, LA. Carvedilol as a protector against the cardiotoxicity induced by anthracyclines (doxorubicin). Revista portuguesa de cardiologia : orgao oficial da Sociedade Portuguesa de Cardiologia = *Portuguese journal of cardiology : an official journal of the Portuguese Society of Cardiology,* 2008, 27, 1277-96.

[92] Oliveira, PJ; Rolo, AP; Sardao, VA; Monteiro, P; Goncalves, L; Providencia, LA, et al. Advantages in the use of carvedilol versus

propranolol for the protection of cardiac mitochondrial function. Revista portuguesa de cardiologia : orgao oficial da Sociedade Portuguesa de Cardiologia = P*ortuguese journal of cardiology : an official journal of the Portuguese Society of Cardiology,* 2004, 23, 1291-8.

[93] Steiner, R; Hellmann, K. Dexrazoxane prevention of anthracycline cardiomyopathy. *Journal of clinical oncology : official journal of the American Society of Clinical Oncology,* 2013, 31, 1379.

[94] Conde-Estevez, D; Mateu-de Antonio, J. *Treatment of anthracycline extravasations using dexrazoxane.* Clinical & translational oncology : official publication of the Federation of Spanish Oncology Societies and of the National Cancer Institute of Mexico, 2013.

[95] Vidall, C; Roe, H; Dougherty, L; Harrold, K. Dexrazoxane: a management option for anthracycline extravasations. *British journal of nursing,* 2013, 22, S6-S12.

[96] Herman, EH; Ferrans, VJ; Myers, CE; Van Vleet, JF. Comparison of the effectiveness of (+/-)-1, 2-bis(3, 5-dioxopiperazinyl-1-yl)propane (ICRF-187) and N-acetylcysteine in preventing chronic doxorubicin cardiotoxicity in beagles. *Cancer research,* 1985, 45, 276-81.

[97] Speyer, JL; Green, MD; Kramer, E; Rey, M; Sanger, J; Ward, C, et al. Protective effect of the bispiperazinedione ICRF-187 against doxorubicin-induced cardiac toxicity in women with advanced breast cancer. *The New England journal of medicine,* 1988, 319, 745-52.

[98] Curran, CF; Narang, PK; Reynolds, RD. Toxicity profile of dexrazoxane (Zinecard, ICRF-187, ADR-529, NSC-169780), a modulator of doxorubicin cardiotoxicity. *Cancer treatment reviews,* 1991, 18, 241-52.

[99] Swain, SM; Whaley, FS; Gerber, MC; Weisberg, S; York, M; Spicer, D, et al. Cardioprotection with dexrazoxane for doxorubicin-containing therapy in advanced breast cancer. *Journal of clinical oncology : official journal of the American Society of Clinical Oncology,* 1997, 15, 1318-32.

[100] Tetef, ML; Synold, TW; Chow, W; Leong, L; Margolin, K; Morgan, R, et al. Phase I trial of 96-hour continuous infusion of dexrazoxane in patients with advanced malignancies. *Clinical cancer research : an official journal of the American Association for Cancer Research,* 2001, 7, 1569-76.

[101] Voest, EE; van Acker, SA; van der Vijgh, WJ; van Asbeck, BS; Bast, A. Comparison of different iron chelators as protective agents against acute

doxorubicin-induced cardiotoxicity. *Journal of molecular and cellular cardiology,* 1994, 26, 1179-85.

[102] Hasinoff, BB; Patel, D; Wu, X. The oral iron chelator ICL670A (deferasirox) does not protect myocytes against doxorubicin. *Free radical biology & medicine,* 2003, 35, 1469-79.

[103] Hasinoff, BB; Herman, EH. Dexrazoxane: how it works in cardiac and tumor cells. Is it a prodrug or is it a drug? *Cardiovascular toxicology,* 2007, 7, 140-4.

[104] Liu, X; Chen, Z; Chua, CC; Ma, YS; Youngberg, GA; Hamdy, R, et al. Melatonin as an effective protector against doxorubicin-induced cardiotoxicity. *American journal of physiology Heart and circulatory physiology,* 2002, 283, H254-63.

[105] Sehested, M; Jensen, PB; Sorensen, BS; Holm, B; Friche, E; Demant, EJ. Antagonistic effect of the cardioprotector (+)-1, 2-bis(3, 5-dioxopiperazinyl-1-yl)propane (ICRF-187) on DNA breaks and cytotoxicity induced by the topoisomerase II directed drugs daunorubicin and etoposide (VP-16). *Biochemical pharmacology,* 1993, 46, 389-93.

[106] Swain, SM; Whaley, FS; Gerber, MC; Ewer, MS; Bianchine, JR; Gams, RA. Delayed administration of dexrazoxane provides cardioprotection for patients with advanced breast cancer treated with doxorubicin-containing therapy. *Journal of clinical oncology : official journal of the American Society of Clinical Oncology,* 1997, 15, 1333-40.

[107] Poljsak, B; Milisav, I. The neglected significance of "antioxidative stress". *Oxidative medicine and cellular longevity,* 2012, 2012, 480895.

[108] Chandran, K; Aggarwal, D; Migrino, RQ; Joseph, J; McAllister, D; Konorev, EA, et al. Doxorubicin inactivates myocardial cytochrome c oxidase in rats: cardioprotection by Mito-Q. *Biophysical journal,* 2009, 96, 1388-98.

[109] Timolati, F; Anliker, T; Groppalli, V; Perriard, JC; Eppenberger, HM; Suter, TM, et al. The role of cell death and myofibrillar damage in contractile dysfunction of long-term cultured adult cardiomyocytes exposed to doxorubicin. *Cytotechnology,* 2009, 61, 25-36.

[110] Lim, CC; Zuppinger, C; Guo, X; Kuster, GM; Helmes, M; Eppenberger, HM, et al. Anthracyclines induce calpain-dependent titin proteolysis and necrosis in cardiomyocytes. *The Journal of biological chemistry,* 2004, 279, 8290-9.

[111] Glembotski, CC. Endoplasmic reticulum stress in the heart. *Circulation research,* 2007, 101, 975-84.

[112] Grune, T; Jung, T; Merker, K; Davies, KJ. Decreased proteolysis caused by protein aggregates, inclusion bodies, plaques, lipofuscin, ceroid, and 'aggresomes' during oxidative stress, aging, and disease. The international journal of biochemistry & cell biology, 2004, 36, 2519-30.
[113] Wang, X; Su, H; Ranek, MJ. Protein quality control and degradation in cardiomyocytes. *Journal of molecular and cellular cardiology,* 2008, 45, 11-27.
[114] Ranek, MJ; Wang, X. Activation of the ubiquitin-proteasome system in doxorubicin cardiomyopathy. *Current hypertension reports,* 2009, 11, 389-95.
[115] Wang, X; Robbins, J. Heart failure and protein quality control. *Circulation research,* 2006, 99, 1315-28.
[116] Patterson, C; Ike, C; Willis, PWt; Stouffer, GA; Willis, MS. The bitter end: the ubiquitin-proteasome system and cardiac dysfunction. *Circulation,* 2007, 115, 1456-63.
[117] Liu, J; Zheng, H; Tang, M; Ryu, YC; Wang, X. A therapeutic dose of doxorubicin activates ubiquitin-proteasome system-mediated proteolysis by acting on both the ubiquitination apparatus and proteasome. *American journal of physiology Heart and circulatory physiology,* 2008, 295, H2541-50.
[118] Sishi, BJ; Loos, B; van Rooyen, J; Engelbrecht, AM. Doxorubicin induces protein ubiquitination and inhibits proteasome activity during cardiotoxicity. *Toxicology,* 2013, 309, 23-9.
[119] Nam, YJ; Mani, K; Wu, L; Peng, CF; Calvert, JW; Foo, RS, et al. The apoptosis inhibitor ARC undergoes ubiquitin-proteasomal-mediated degradation in response to death stimuli: identification of a degradation-resistant mutant. *The Journal of biological chemistry*, 2007, 282, 5522-8.
[120] Fukuda, N; Sasaki, D; Ishiwata, S; Kurihara, S. Length dependence of tension generation in rat skinned cardiac muscle: role of titin in the Frank-Starling mechanism of the heart. *Circulation,* 2001, 104, 1639-45.
[121] Haq, S; Michael, A; Andreucci, M; Bhattacharya, K; Dotto, P; Walters, B, et al. Stabilization of beta-catenin by a Wnt-independent mechanism regulates cardiomyocyte growth. *Proceedings of the National Academy of Sciences of the United States of America,* 2003, 100, 4610-5.
[122] Yamamoto, Y; Hoshino, Y; Ito, T; Nariai, T; Mohri, T; Obana, M, et al. Atrogin-1 ubiquitin ligase is upregulated by doxorubicin via p38-MAP kinase in cardiac myocytes. *Cardiovascular research,* 2008, 79, 89-96.

[123] Li, HH; Kedar, V; Zhang, C; McDonough, H; Arya, R; Wang, DZ, et al. Atrogin-1/muscle atrophy F-box inhibits calcineurin-dependent cardiac hypertrophy by participating in an SCF ubiquitin ligase complex. *The Journal of clinical investigation, 2004*, 114, 1058-71.

[124] Murton, AJ; Constantin, D; Greenhaff, PL. The involvement of the ubiquitin proteasome system in human skeletal muscle remodelling and atrophy. *Biochimica et biophysica acta,* 2008, 1782, 730-43.

[125] Kalivendi, SV; Konorev, EA; Cunningham, S; Vanamala, SK; Kaji, EH; Joseph, J, et al. Doxorubicin activates nuclear factor of activated T-lymphocytes and Fas ligand transcription: role of mitochondrial reactive oxygen species and calcium. *The Biochemical journal,* 2005, 389, 527-39.

[126] Ito, T; Fujio, Y; Takahashi, K; Azuma, J. Degradation of NFAT5, a transcriptional regulator of osmotic stress-related genes, is a critical event for doxorubicin-induced cytotoxicity in cardiac myocytes. *The Journal of biological chemistry, 2007*, 282, 1152-60.

[127] Ito, T; Fujio, Y; Schaffer, SW; Azuma, J. Involvement of transcriptional factor TonEBP in the regulation of the taurine transporter in the cardiomyocyte. *Advances in experimental medicine and biology,* 2009, 643, 523-32.

[128] LoConte, NK; Thomas, JP; Alberti, D; Heideman, J; Binger, K; Marnocha, R, et al. A phase I pharmacodynamic trial of bortezomib in combination with doxorubicin in patients with advanced cancer. *Cancer chemotherapy and pharmacology,* 2008, 63, 109-15.

[129] Umlauf, J; Horky, M. Molecular biology of doxorubicin-induced cardiomyopathy. *Experimental and clinical cardiology,* 2002, 7, 35-9.

[130] Murphy, AM; Thompson, WR; Peng, LF; Jones, L, 2nd. Regulation of the rat cardiac troponin I gene by the transcription factor GATA-4. *The Biochemical journal,* 1997, 322 (Pt 2), 393-401.

[131] Kim, Y; Ma, AG; Kitta, K; Fitch, SN; Ikeda, T; Ihara, Y, et al. Anthracycline-induced suppression of GATA-4 transcription factor: implication in the regulation of cardiac myocyte apoptosis. *Molecular pharmacology,* 2003, 63, 368-77.

[132] Aries, A; Paradis, P; Lefebvre, C; Schwartz, RJ; Nemer, M. Essential role of GATA-4 in cell survival and drug-induced cardiotoxicity. *Proceedings of the National Academy of Sciences of the United States of America,* 2004, 101, 6975-80.

[133] Yi, X; Bekeredjian, R; DeFilippis, NJ; Siddiquee, Z; Fernandez, E; Shohet, RV. Transcriptional analysis of doxorubicin-induced

cardiotoxicity. *American journal of physiology Heart and circulatory physiology,* 2006, 290, H1098-102.
[134] Jeyaseelan, R; Poizat, C; Baker, RK; Abdishoo, S; Isterabadi, LB; Lyons, GE, et al. A novel cardiac-restricted target for doxorubicin. CARP, a nuclear modulator of gene expression in cardiac progenitor cells and cardiomyocytes. *The Journal of biological chemistry, 1997,* 272, 22800-8.
[135] Zordoky, BN; Anwar-Mohamed, A; Aboutabl, ME; El-Kadi, AO. Acute doxorubicin cardiotoxicity alters cardiac cytochrome P450 expression and arachidonic acid metabolism in rats. *Toxicology and applied pharmacology,* 2010, 242, 38-46.
[136] Sayed-Ahmed, MM; Al-Shabanah, OA; Hafez, MM; Aleisa, AM; Al-Rejaie, SS. Inhibition of gene expression of heart fatty acid binding protein and organic cation/carnitine transporter in doxorubicin cardiomyopathic rat model. *European journal of pharmacology,* 2010, 640, 143-9.
[137] Pointon, AV; Walker, TM; Phillips, KM; Luo, J; Riley, J; Zhang, SD, et al. Doxorubicin in vivo rapidly alters expression and translation of myocardial electron transport chain genes, leads to ATP loss and caspase 3 activation. *PloS one,* 2010, 5, e12733.
[138] Arai, M; Tomaru, K; Takizawa, T; Sekiguchi, K; Yokoyama, T; Suzuki, T, et al. Sarcoplasmic reticulum genes are selectively down-regulated in cardiomyopathy produced by doxorubicin in rabbits. *Journal of molecular and cellular cardiology*, 1998, 30, 243-54.
[139] Jeyaseelan, R; Poizat, C; Wu, HY; Kedes, L. Molecular mechanisms of doxorubicin-induced cardiomyopathy. Selective suppression of Reiske iron-sulfur protein, ADP/ATP translocase, and phosphofructokinase genes is associated with ATP depletion in rat cardiomyocytes. *The Journal of biological chemistry,* 1997, 272, 5828-32.
[140] Maeda, A; Honda, M; Kuramochi, T; Takabatake, T. Doxorubicin cardiotoxicity: diastolic cardiac myocyte dysfunction as a result of impaired calcium handling in isolated cardiac myocytes. *Japanese circulation journal,* 1998, 62, 505-11.
[141] Maejima, Y; Adachi, S; Ito, H; Hirao, K; Isobe, M. Induction of premature senescence in cardiomyocytes by doxorubicin as a novel mechanism of myocardial damage. *Aging cell,* 2008, 7, 125-36.
[142] Kajstura, J; Rota, M; Urbanek, K; Hosoda, T; Bearzi, C; Anversa, P, et al. The telomere-telomerase axis and the heart. *Antioxidants & redox signaling,* 2006, 8, 2125-41.

[143] Bernhard, D; Laufer, G. The aging cardiomyocyte: a mini-review. *Gerontology,* 2008, 54, 24-31.

[144] Willerson, JT; Ridker, PM. Inflammation as a cardiovascular risk factor. *Circulation, 2004*, 109, II2-10.

[145] Mann, DL. Inflammatory mediators and the failing heart: past, present, and the foreseeable future. *Circulation research,* 2002, 91, 988-98.

[146] Bujak, M; Frangogiannis, NG. The role of IL-1 in the pathogenesis of heart disease. *Archivum immunologiae et therapiae experimentalis,* 2009, 57, 165-76.

[147] Guo, RM; Xu, WM; Lin, JC; Mo, LQ; Hua, XX; Chen, PX, et al. Activation of the p38 MAPK/NF-kappaB pathway contributes to doxorubicin-induced inflammation and cytotoxicity in H9c2 cardiac cells. *Molecular medicine reports,* 2013, 8, 603-8.

[148] Zhu, J; Zhang, J; Zhang, L; Du, R; Xiang, D; Wu, M, et al. Interleukin-1 signaling mediates acute doxorubicin-induced cardiotoxicity. *Biomedicine & pharmacotherapy = Biomedecine & pharmacotherapie,* 2011, 65, 481-5.

[149] Zhu, J; Zhang, J; Xiang, D; Zhang, Z; Zhang, L; Wu, M, et al. Recombinant human interleukin-1 receptor antagonist protects mice against acute doxorubicin-induced cardiotoxicity. *European journal of pharmacology,* 2010, 643, 247-53.

[150] Dunne, A; O'Neill, LA. The interleukin-1 receptor/Toll-like receptor superfamily: signal transduction during inflammation and host defense. *Science's STKE : signal transduction knowledge environment,* 2003, 2003, re3.

[151] Mann, DL; Topkara, VK; Evans, S; Barger, PM. Innate immunity in the adult mammalian heart: for whom the cell tolls. *Transactions of the American Clinical and Climatological Association,* 2010, 121, 34-50; discussion -1.

[152] Riad, A; Bien, S; Gratz, M; Escher, F; Westermann, D; Heimesaat, MM, et al. Toll-like receptor-4 deficiency attenuates doxorubicin-induced cardiomyopathy in mice. *European journal of heart failure,* 2008, 10, 233-43.

[153] Nozaki, N; Shishido, T; Takeishi, Y; Kubota, I. Modulation of doxorubicin-induced cardiac dysfunction in toll-like receptor-2-knockout mice. *Circulation,* 2004, 110, 2869-74.

[154] Sakata, Y; Dong, JW; Vallejo, JG; Huang, CH; Baker, JS; Tracey, KJ, et al. Toll-like receptor 2 modulates left ventricular function following

ischemia-reperfusion injury. *American journal of physiology Heart and circulatory physiology,* 2007, 292, H503-9.

[155] Shishido, T; Nozaki, N; Yamaguchi, S; Shibata, Y; Nitobe, J; Miyamoto, T, et al. Toll-like receptor-2 modulates ventricular remodeling after myocardial infarction. *Circulation,* 2003, 108, 2905-10.

[156] Frantz, S; Kelly, RA; Bourcier, T. Role of TLR-2 in the activation of nuclear factor kappaB by oxidative stress in cardiac myocytes. *The Journal of biological chemistry, 2001*, 276, 5197-203.

[157] Wang, S; Kotamraju, S; Konorev, E; Kalivendi, S; Joseph, J; Kalyanaraman, B. Activation of nuclear factor-kappaB during doxorubicin-induced apoptosis in endothelial cells and myocytes is pro-apoptotic: the role of hydrogen peroxide. *The Biochemical journal,* 2002, 367, 729-40.

[158] Timmers, L; Sluijter, JP; van Keulen, JK; Hoefer, IE; Nederhoff, MG; Goumans, MJ, et al. Toll-like receptor 4 mediates maladaptive left ventricular remodeling and impairs cardiac function after myocardial infarction. *Circulation research,* 2008, 102, 257-64.

[159] Zhang, YW; Shi, J; Li, YJ; Wei, L. *Cardiomyocyte death in doxorubicin-induced cardiotoxicity. Archivum immunologiae et therapiae experimentalis,* 2009, 57, 435-45.

[160] Arola, OJ; Saraste, A; Pulkki, K; Kallajoki, M; Parvinen, M; Voipio-Pulkki, LM. Acute doxorubicin cardiotoxicity involves cardiomyocyte apoptosis. *Cancer research,* 2000, 60, 1789-92.

[161] Kotamraju, S; Konorev, EA; Joseph, J; Kalyanaraman, B. Doxorubicin-induced apoptosis in endothelial cells and cardiomyocytes is ameliorated by nitrone spin traps and ebselen. Role of reactive oxygen and nitrogen species. *The Journal of biological chemistry,* 2000, 275, 33585-92.

[162] Bennink, RJ; van den Hoff, MJ; van Hemert, FJ; de Bruin, KM; Spijkerboer, AL; Vanderheyden, JL, et al. Annexin V imaging of acute doxorubicin cardiotoxicity (apoptosis) in rats. *Journal of nuclear medicine : official publication, Society of Nuclear Medicine,* 2004, 45, 842-8.

[163] Kawamura, T; Hasegawa, K; Morimoto, T; Iwai-Kanai, E; Miyamoto, S; Kawase, Y, et al. Expression of p300 protects cardiac myocytes from apoptosis in vivo. *Biochemical and biophysical research communications*, 2004, 315, 733-8.

[164] Fisher, PW; Salloum, F; Das, A; Hyder, H; Kukreja, RC. Phosphodiesterase-5 inhibition with sildenafil attenuates cardiomyocyte apoptosis and left ventricular dysfunction in a chronic model of doxorubicin cardiotoxicity. *Circulation,* 2005, 111, 1601-10.

[165] Wang, GW; Klein, JB; Kang, YJ. Metallothionein inhibits doxorubicin-induced mitochondrial cytochrome c release and caspase-3 activation in cardiomyocytes. *The Journal of pharmacology and experimental therapeutics,* 2001, 298, 461-8.

[166] Childs, AC; Phaneuf, SL; Dirks, AJ; Phillips, T; Leeuwenburgh, C. Doxorubicin treatment in vivo causes cytochrome C release and cardiomyocyte apoptosis, as well as increased mitochondrial efficiency, superoxide dismutase activity, and Bcl-2:Bax ratio. *Cancer research,* 2002, 62, 4592-8.

[167] Deniaud, A; Sharaf el dein, O; Maillier, E; Poncet, D; Kroemer, G; Lemaire, C, et al. Endoplasmic reticulum stress induces calcium-dependent permeability transition, mitochondrial outer membrane permeabilization and apoptosis. *Oncogene,* 2008, 27, 285-99.

[168] L'Ecuyer, T; Sanjeev, S; Thomas, R; Novak, R; Das, L; Campbell, W, et al. DNA damage is an early event in doxorubicin-induced cardiac myocyte death. *American journal of physiology Heart and circulatory physiology,* 2006, 291, H1273-80.

[169] Liu, X; Chua, CC; Gao, J; Chen, Z; Landy, CL; Hamdy, R, et al. Pifithrin-alpha protects against doxorubicin-induced apoptosis and acute cardiotoxicity in mice. *American journal of physiology Heart and circulatory physiology,* 2004, 286, H933-9.

[170] Sardao, VA; Oliveira, PJ; Holy, J; Oliveira, CR; Wallace, KB. Doxorubicin-induced mitochondrial dysfunction is secondary to nuclear p53 activation in H9c2 cardiomyoblasts. *Cancer chemotherapy and pharmacology,* 2009, 64, 811-27.

[171] Suliman, HB; Carraway, MS; Ali, AS; Reynolds, CM; Welty-Wolf, KE; Piantadosi, CA. The CO/HO system reverses inhibition of mitochondrial biogenesis and prevents murine doxorubicin cardiomyopathy. *The Journal of clinical investigation,* 2007, 117, 3730-41.

[172] Fan, GC; Zhou, X; Wang, X; Song, G; Qian, J; Nicolaou, P, et al. Heat shock protein 20 interacting with phosphorylated Akt reduces doxorubicin-triggered oxidative stress and cardiotoxicity. *Circulation research,* 2008, 103, 1270-9.

[173] Nakamura, T; Ueda, Y; Juan, Y; Katsuda, S; Takahashi, H; Koh, E. Fas-mediated apoptosis in adriamycin-induced cardiomyopathy in rats: In vivo study. *Circulation,* 2000, 102, 572-8.

[174] Niu, J; Azfer, A; Wang, K; Wang, X; Kolattukudy, PE. Cardiac-targeted expression of soluble fas attenuates doxorubicin-induced cardiotoxicity in mice. *The Journal of pharmacology and experimental therapeutics,* 2009, 328, 740-8.

[175] Ikegami, E; Fukazawa, R; Kanbe, M; Watanabe, M; Abe, M; Watanabe, M, et al. Edaravone, a potent free radical scavenger, prevents anthracycline-induced myocardial cell death. *Circulation journal : official journal of the Japanese Circulation Society,* 2007, 71, 1815-20.

[176] Riad, A; Bien, S; Westermann, D; Becher, PM; Loya, K; Landmesser, U, et al. Pretreatment with statin attenuates the cardiotoxicity of Doxorubicin in mice. *Cancer research,* 2009, 69, 695-9.

[177] Casey, TM; Arthur, PG; Bogoyevitch, MA. Necrotic death without mitochondrial dysfunction-delayed death of cardiac myocytes following oxidative stress. *Biochimica et biophysica acta,* 2007, 1773, 342-51.

[178] Sishi, BJ; Loos, B; van Rooyen, J; Engelbrecht, AM. Autophagy upregulation promotes survival and attenuates doxorubicin-induced cardiotoxicity. *Biochemical pharmacology,* 2013, 85, 124-34.

[179] An, T; Huang, Y; Zhou, Q; Wei, BQ; Zhang, RC; Yin, SJ, et al. Neuregulin-1 attenuates doxorubicin-induced autophagy in neonatal rat cardiomyocytes. *Journal of cardiovascular pharmacology,* 2013, 62, 130-7.

[180] Dimitrakis, P; Romay-Ogando, MI; Timolati, F; Suter, TM; Zuppinger, C. Effects of doxorubicin cancer therapy on autophagy and the ubiquitin-proteasome system in long-term cultured adult rat cardiomyocytes. *Cell and tissue research,* 2012, 350, 361-72.

[181] Hoyer-Hansen, M; Bastholm, L; Szyniarowski, P; Campanella, M; Szabadkai, G; Farkas, T, et al. *Control of macroautophagy by calcium, calmodulin-dependent kinase kinase-beta, and Bcl-2. Molecular cell,* 2007, 25, 193-205.

[182] Maiuri, MC; Zalckvar, E; Kimchi, A; Kroemer, G. Self-eating and self-killing: crosstalk between autophagy and apoptosis. *Nature reviews Molecular cell biology,* 2007, 8, 741-52.

[183] Nishida, K; Kyoi, S; Yamaguchi, O; Sadoshima, J; Otsu, K. The role of autophagy in the heart. *Cell death and differentiation,* 2009, 16, 31-8.

[184] Nishida, K; Yamaguchi, O; Otsu, K. Crosstalk between autophagy and apoptosis in heart disease. *Circulation research,* 2008, 103, 343-51.

[185] Terman, A; Gustafsson, B; Brunk, UT. The lysosomal-mitochondrial axis theory of postmitotic aging and cell death. *Chemico-biological interactions, 2006*, 163, 29-37.
[186] Green, PS; Leeuwenburgh, C. Mitochondrial dysfunction is an early indicator of doxorubicin-induced apoptosis. *Biochimica et biophysica acta,* 2002, 1588, 94-101.
[187] Jang, YM; Kendaiah, S; Drew, B; Phillips, T; Selman, C; Julian, D, et al. Doxorubicin treatment in vivo activates caspase-12 mediated cardiac apoptosis in both male and female rats. *FEBS letters,* 2004, 577, 483-90.
[188] Shapira, J; Gotfried, M; Lishner, M; Ravid, M. Reduced cardiotoxicity of doxorubicin by a 6-hour infusion regimen. A prospective randomized evaluation. *Cancer,* 1990, 65, 870-3.
[189] Legha, SS; Benjamin, RS; Mackay, B; Ewer, M; Wallace, S; Valdivieso, M, et al. Reduction of doxorubicin cardiotoxicity by prolonged continuous intravenous infusion. *Annals of internal medicine,* 1982, 96, 133-9.
[190] Bielack, SS; Erttmann, R; Winkler, K; Landbeck, G. Doxorubicin: effect of different schedules on toxicity and anti-tumor efficacy. *European journal of cancer & clinical oncology*, 1989, 25, 873-82.
[191] Berrak, SG; Ewer, MS; Jaffe, N; Pearson, P; Ried, H; Zietz, HA, et al. Doxorubicin cardiotoxicity in children: reduced incidence of cardiac dysfunction associated with continuous-infusion schedules. *Oncology reports,* 2001, 8, 611-4.
[192] Lipshultz, SE; Giantris, AL; Lipsitz, SR; Kimball Dalton, V; Asselin, BL; Barr, RD, et al. Doxorubicin administration by continuous infusion is not cardioprotective: the Dana-Farber 91-01 Acute Lymphoblastic Leukemia protocol. *Journal of clinical oncology : official journal of the American Society of Clinical Oncology*, 2002, 20, 1677-82.
[193] Gabizon, AA; Lyass, O; Berry, GJ; Wildgust, M. Cardiac safety of pegylated liposomal doxorubicin (Doxil/Caelyx) demonstrated by endomyocardial biopsy in patients with advanced malignancies. *Cancer investigation,* 2004, 22, 663-9.
[194] O'Brien, ME; Wigler, N; Inbar, M; Rosso, R; Grischke, E; Santoro, A, et al. Reduced cardiotoxicity and comparable efficacy in a phase III trial of pegylated liposomal doxorubicin HCl (CAELYX/Doxil) versus conventional doxorubicin for first-line treatment of metastatic breast cancer. *Annals of oncology : official journal of the European Society for Medical Oncology / ESMO,* 2004, 15, 440-9.

[195] Nagykalnai, T. [Non-pegylated doxorubicin (Myocet(R)) as the less cardiotoxic alternative of free doxorubicin*]. Magyar onkologia,* 2010, 54, 359-67.

[196] Harris, L; Batist, G; Belt, R; Rovira, D; Navari, R; Azarnia, N, et al. Liposome-encapsulated doxorubicin compared with conventional doxorubicin in a randomized multicenter trial as first-line therapy of metastatic breast carcinoma. *Cancer, 2002*, 94, 25-36.

[197] Juliano, RL; Stamp, D. The effect of particle size and charge on the clearance rates of liposomes and liposome encapsulated drugs. *Biochemical and biophysical research communications,* 1975, 63, 651-8.

[198] Poste, G; Bucana, C; Raz, A; Bugelski, P; Kirsh, R; Fidler, IJ. Analysis of the fate of systemically administered liposomes and implications for their use in drug delivery. *Cancer research,* 1982, 42, 1412-22.

[199] Gabizon, A; Shmeeda, H; Barenholz, Y. Pharmacokinetics of pegylated liposomal Doxorubicin: review of animal and human studies. *Clinical pharmacokinetics,* 2003, 42, 419-36.

[200] Safra, T; Muggia, F; Jeffers, S; Tsao-Wei, DD; Groshen, S; Lyass, O, et al. Pegylated liposomal doxorubicin (doxil): reduced clinical cardiotoxicity in patients reaching or exceeding cumulative doses of 500 mg/m2. *Annals of oncology : official journal of the European Society for Medical Oncology / ESMO,* 2000, 11, 1029-33.

[201] Judson, I; Radford, JA; Harris, M; Blay, JY; van Hoesel, Q; le Cesne, A, et al. Randomised phase II trial of pegylated liposomal doxorubicin (DOXIL/CAELYX) versus doxorubicin in the treatment of advanced or metastatic soft tissue sarcoma: a study by the EORTC Soft Tissue and Bone Sarcoma Group. *European journal of cancer,* 2001, 37, 870-7.

[202] de la Fouchardiere, C; Largillier, R; Goubely, Y; Hardy-Bessard, AC; Slama, B; Cretin, J, et al. Docetaxel and pegylated liposomal doxorubicin combination as first-line therapy for metastatic breast cancer patients: results of the phase II GINECO trial CAPYTTOLE. *Annals of oncology : official journal of the European Society for Medical Oncology / ESMO,* 2009, 20, 1959-63.

[203] Morabito, A; Gattuso, D; Stani, SC; Fanelli, M; Ferrau, F; De Sio, L, et al. Safety and activity of the combination of pegylated liposomal doxorubicin and weekly docetaxel in advanced breast cancer. *Breast cancer research and treatment,* 2004, 86, 249-57.

[204] Alexopoulos, A; Karamouzis, MV; Stavrinides, H; Ardavanis, A; Kandilis, K; Stavrakakis, J, et al. Phase II study of pegylated liposomal

doxorubicin (Caelyx) and docetaxel as first-line treatment in metastatic breast cancer. *Annals of oncology : official journal of the European Society for Medical Oncology / ESMO,* 2004, 15, 891-5.

[205] Lyass, O; Uziely, B; Ben-Yosef, R; Tzemach, D; Heshing, NI; Lotem, M, et al. Correlation of toxicity with pharmacokinetics of pegylated liposomal doxorubicin (Doxil) in metastatic breast carcinoma. *Cancer,* 2000, 89, 1037-47.

[206] Briasoulis, E; Karavasilis, V; Tzamakou, E; Rammou, D; Soulti, K; Piperidou, C, et al. Interaction pharmacokinetics of pegylated liposomal doxorubicin (Caelyx) on coadministration with paclitaxel or docetaxel. *Cancer chemotherapy and pharmacology,* 2004, 53, 452-7.

[207] Batist, G; Ramakrishnan, G; Rao, CS; Chandrasekharan, A; Gutheil, J; Guthrie, T, et al. Reduced cardiotoxicity and preserved antitumor efficacy of liposome-encapsulated doxorubicin and cyclophosphamide compared with conventional doxorubicin and cyclophosphamide in a randomized, multicenter trial of metastatic breast cancer. *Journal of clinical oncology : official journal of the American Society of Clinical Oncology,* 2001, 19, 1444-54.

[208] Mitra, S; Gaur, U; Ghosh, PC; Maitra, AN. Tumour targeted delivery of encapsulated dextran-doxorubicin conjugate using chitosan nanoparticles as carrier. *Journal of controlled release : official journal of the Controlled Release Society,* 2001, 74, 317-23.

[209] Sun, K; Wang, J; Zhang, J; Hua, M; Liu, C; Chen, T. Dextran-g-PEI nanoparticles as a carrier for co-delivery of adriamycin and plasmid into osteosarcoma cells. *International journal of biological macromolecules,* 2011, 49, 173-80.

[210] Tan, ML; Friedhuber, AM; Dunstan, DE; Choong, PF; Dass, CR. The performance of doxorubicin encapsulated in chitosan-dextran sulphate microparticles in an osteosarcoma model. *Biomaterials,* 2010, 31, 541-51.

[211] Jain, KK; Casper, ES; Geller, NL; Hakes, TB; Kaufman, RJ; Currie, V, et al. A prospective randomized comparison of epirubicin and doxorubicin in patients with advanced breast cancer. *Journal of clinical oncology : official journal of the American Society of Clinical Oncology,* 1985, 3, 818-26.

[212] Brambilla, C; Rossi, A; Bonfante, V; Ferrari, L; Villani, F; Crippa, F, et al. Phase II study of doxorubicin versus epirubicin in advanced breast cancer. *Cancer treatment reports,* 1986, 70, 261-6.

[213] Robert, J; Vrignaud, P; Nguyen-Ngoc, T; Iliadis, A; Mauriac, L; Hurteloup, P. Comparative pharmacokinetics and metabolism of doxorubicin and epirubicin in patients with metastatic breast cancer. *Cancer treatment reports,* 1985, 69, 633-40.

[214] Burnell, M; Levine, MN; Chapman, JA; Bramwell, V; Gelmon, K; Walley, B, et al. Cyclophosphamide, epirubicin, and Fluorouracil versus dose-dense epirubicin and cyclophosphamide followed by Paclitaxel versus Doxorubicin and cyclophosphamide followed by Paclitaxel in node-positive or high-risk node-negative breast cancer. *Journal of clinical oncology : official journal of the American Society of Clinical Oncology*, 2010, 28, 77-82.

[215] Khasraw, M; Bell, R; Dang, C. Epirubicin: is it like doxorubicin in breast cancer? A clinical review. *Breast,* 2012, 21, 142-9.

[216] Ryberg, M; Nielsen, D; Skovsgaard, T; Hansen, J; Jensen, BV; Dombernowsky, P. Epirubicin cardiotoxicity: an analysis of 469 patients with metastatic breast cancer. *Journal of clinical oncology : official journal of the American Society of Clinical Oncology,* 1998, 16, 3502-8.

In: Doxorubicin
Editor: Melinda Pache

ISBN: 978-1-63117-233-5

Chapter 4

ADVANCED THERAPIES OF DOXORUBICIN BY CARRIER OF DRUG DELIVERY SYSTEM OR COMBINED FOOD COMPONENTS

Yasuyuki Sadzuka *
School of Pharmacy, Iwate Medical University,
Shiwa-Gun, Iwate, Japan

ABSTRACT

Doxorubicin (DOX) is classical but useful antitumor agent. DOX is used for the treatment of a variety of malignancies including solid tumors and leukemia due to its broad spectrum antitumor activity. However, DOX-induced cardiac toxicity as its adverse reaction is a dose limiting factor. Namely, DOX has double-edged effect with utilized action and severe adverse reaction. To make the most of ability of DOX, it is necessary to advance its therapy.

One of the advanced therapies is treatment of liposomal DOX. Liposomes are the principal means of effectively using medicines and are broadly recognized as a drug delivery system (DDS) carrier. However, liposomes after intravenous injection are rapidly taken up by reticuloendothelial system (RES) cells in the liver and spleen. This phenomenon reduces the effectiveness of liposomes as a drug carrier. Therefore, techniques for avoiding catch by RES cells and increasing the effectivity of liposomes based on polyethyleneglycol (PEG) modification

* Professor. E-mail : ysadzuka@iwate-med.ac.jp.

on the surface of liposomes have been developed. DOX entrapped liposome by PEG modification induced an increase in the DOX level in the plasma and tumor and a decrease in this level in the liver. In vitro, The high entrapped amount of DOX into liposome demonstrated the usefulness of DOX liposomes for tumor cell uptake. Furthermore, anchor length of PEG-lipid on liposomal surface was clarified to be important on liposomal DOX uptake into tumor cell. The therapeutic index on peritoneal dissemination was influenced by particle size of liposomal DOX. The efficacy of liposomal DOX by modification using a mixture of PEG2000 and PEG with short PEG-chain was superior.

Another advanced therapy is biochemical modulation by foods or their components, not combined medicines. Theanine (specific amino acid in green tea) significantly enhanced the inhibitory effect of DOX on tumor growth and increased the DOX concentration in the tumor, and then the oral administration of theanine or green tea similarly enhanced the antitumor activity of DOX. Moreover, the combined theanine with DOX suppressed the hepatic metastasis of ovarian sarcoma. It was revealed that these effects by theanine were novel mechanism of enhancement of antitumor efficacy of DOX via the inhibition of glutamate transporters.

Anserine (a dipeptide contained in fowl and migratory fish) was increased DOX induced antitumor activity with the elevation of DOX concentration in the tumor. Anserine considered to take into tumor cells via a dipeptide transporter, and it resulted in an increase of the DOX influx in tumor cells. Taurine (a major amino acid in fish and meat) and cucurbitacin E and I (a bitter tasting component of squash fruit) co-treatment was confirmed to increase DOX induced antitumor activity without an increase in adverse reactions by DOX, too. Namely, it was clarified that some foods and their components were useful as a modulator to enhance the therapeutic index of cancer patients and improve quality of life.

In conclusion, advanced therapies of DOX by liposomalization of DOX or combined food components with DOX was expected to contribute to cancer chemotherapy.

1. Introduction

Doxorubicin (DOX) is used for the treatment of a variety of malignancies such as solid tumors and leukemia due to its broad antitumor activity spectrum. The mechanism underlying the antitumor activity and cytotoxic effect of DOX has been proposed to be the inhibitions of DNA polymerase and topoisomerase II [1]. In contrast, the clinical use of DOX is restricted by severe adverse reactions [2,3]. Cardiotoxicity as dose limiting factor is a major adverse reaction of DOX involved in free radical reactions mediated by DOX in the heart [4-6]. Namely, DOX has double-edged effect with utilized action and severe adverse reactions.

Furthermore, the antitumor activity of DOX depends on its concentration in the tumor cells, namely, the antitumor activity of DOX can be enhanced by increasing the DOX concentration in the tumor cells. In multidrug resistant tumor cells, an active efflux pump overexpressed on the plasma membrane induces a reduction of the antitumor activity of DOX by enhancing the efflux of DOX from tumor cells [7-11]. Attempts on reversal of multidrug resistant tumor cells by suppressing the efflux pump were made [12-19]. However, these attempts might increase DOX induced adverse reaction by the suppression of these efflux pumps on the normal cells. Thus, to make the most of ability of DOX, it is necessary to improve its therapy.

In this review, advanced therapies of doxorubicin by carrier of drug delivery system or combined food components were described.

2. Liposome as a Drug Delivery System

Liposomes are the principal means of effectively using medicines and are broadly recognized as a drug delivery system (DDS) carrier. However, liposomes after intravenous injection are rapidly taken up by reticuloendothelial system (RES) cells in the liver and spleen. This phenomenon reduces the effectiveness of liposomes as a drug carrier. Therefore, techniques for avoiding catch by RES cells and increasing the effectivity of liposomes based on polyethyleneglycol (PEG) modification on the surface of liposomes have been developed. DOX entrapped liposome by PEG modification induced an increase in the DOX level in the plasma and tumor and a decrease in this level in the liver. In this section, the effects of entrapped amount of DOX into liposome, anchor length of PEG-lipid on liposomal surface and particle size of liposomal DOX on tumor cell uptake, and the therapeutic index on peritoneal dissemination were clarified. Furthermore, it is suggested that the efficacy of liposomal DOX by modification using a mixture of PEG2000 and PEG with short PEG-chain was superior.

2.1. Tumor Cell Uptake of DOX-Contained Liposome

DOX after intravenous injection immediately disappears in the blood [20-24] but causes severe bone marrow suppression and cardiotoxicity [25,26]. Therefore, because DOX has a strong antitumor effect and severe adverse reaction, it was also one of the drugs used in the most advanced studies on liposomalization [27-29]. It is known that the tissue distribution of liposomes is dominated by the entrapped drug, the lipid composition of the liposomes and the physical properties of the liposomes.

DOX (1.0 or 0.6 or 0.2 mg/26 μmol lipid) entrapped liposomes (dimyristoylphosphatidyl- choline (DMPC): cholesterol: dimyristoyl-phosphatidylglycerol (DMPG) = 100 : 100 : 60) were prepared (DM1.0, DM0.6, DM0.2), according to a modification [29] of the method of Bangham [30]. After administration of these liposomes with the same dose of DOX and different doses of lipid, there was no difference in the tissue distribution of DOX with a change in the amount of DOX entrapped in the liposomes. In contrast, after the administration of DOX entrapping liposome contained distearoylphosphatidylcholine (DSPC) by using DSPC instead of DMPC (DS1.0, DS0.6 and DS0.2), an increase in the amount of DOX entrapped in the liposomes induced an increase in the DOX concentrations in the plasma and tumor and a decrease in the DOX concentration in the liver. The order of the plasma levels of DOX was DS0.2 < DS0.6 = DS1.0. Furthermore, an increase in the entrapped amount in the liposomes increased the DOX concentration in tumor and the DOX concentration after DS1.0 administration was 4.9 fold ($P < 0.001$) that after DOX solution treatment [31]. It is suggested that the increase in the DOX level per amount of the lipid comprising the liposomes increased the usefulness of liposomalization in vivo.

The high entrapped amount, which exhibited good quality in vivo, was also useful for the tumor cell uptake of DOX liposome in vitro. It appeared that in relation to the tumor cell uptake in vitro, the DOX liposome could be divided into a low uptake group (DS0.6 and DS0.2) and a high uptake group (DS2.0 and DS1.0). It was considered that in the case of the low uptake group, as many of the liposomes were unable to enter the tumor cells due to the lipid saturation of the tumor cells. On the other hand, in the high uptake group with the same concentration of DOX, the lipid concentration in the medium decreased with an increase in the amount of DOX entrapped in the liposomes. It is expected that the cell uptake of DOX-containing liposomes would dependently increase with the number of liposomes and the increase in the amount of DOX entrapped in the liposomes would induced an increase in the tumor cell uptake of DOX-containing liposomes. This speculation has been supported by the finding that the addition of empty liposomes to DM1.0 and DS1.0 liposome suspensions decreased the DOX uptake by the tumor cells to 62 % and 38 %, respectively. These phenomena in vitro were also observed in vivo.

Using DSPC liposomes which appeared superior as to the tissue distribution, the antitumor activity after the administrations of DS2.0 (high uptake by tumor cells in vitro) and DS0.6 (low uptake) were examined. As judged from the tumor weight, the DOX induced antitumor activity increased with an increase in the entrapped amount. Furthermore, this effect was supported by the DOX concentration in the tumor. Thus, the higher amount of DOX entrapped in liposomes has been confirmed to be beneficial in vitro and in vivo.

The modification of the liposomal surface with some PEG-lipids has produced good results in terms of a prolonged circulation in the blood, but it is apprehensive to be a danger that modification of the liposomal surface with some PEG-lipids prevents the connection of liposome and tumor cell by the existence of macromolecules on the liposomal surface [32]. Next, the effect of modification of the liposomal surface with PEG-lipids by changing the PEG chain length and anchor length, on liposome uptake into tumor cells were examined. The uptake of DOX in liposomal DOX (LDOX) and PEG-LDOX groups by tumor cells showed a time-dependent increase [33]. In addition, PEG-LDOX increased uptake of DOX more than LDOX in vitro, which indicated the PEG-LDOX escaped from the cells of the RES such as the liver and spleen by avoiding adhesion to opsonin and were distributed to tumor cells by passive targeting on uptake of DOX into tumor cells in vivo.

The longer PEG chain length in PEG-dimyristoylglycerol (PEG-DMG) modified liposome (PM-LDOX) and PEG-distearoylglycerol (PEG-DSG) modified liposome (PS-LDOX) groups increased tumor cell uptake of DOX. In contrast, PEG-dipalmytoylglycerol (PEG-DPG) modified liposome (PP-LDOX) had the greatest uptake, at 2.5 fold and 5.1 fold the level of PM-LDOX and PS-LDOX, respectively. The uptake of DOX in PP-LDOX (PEG2000) group exceeded that in PM-LDOX (PEG5000) and PS-LDOX (PEG5000). Hence, the cell uptake of DOX did not only depend on the length of PEG chain alone. With these PEG-liposome, there was little change in particle size, surface electric potential, and cmc, but there was change in octanol/water of PEG-lipid. So, the balance between the length of the PEG chain and the length of the anchor was important.

The less PEG-lipid with longer the anchor length incorporated into liposomes. However, there was no correlation with cell uptake of DOX and modifying amount of PEG-lipid, suggesting that the effect of cell uptake of DOX into tumor cells was caused by factors other than the modifying amount of PEG. In contrast, the difference in the modified stability of PEG-lipids in the liposomal surface in serum is important. When the polar head group was PEG2000, the order of residual ratio of PEG-lipid on liposomal membrane was PEG-palmytoyl > PEG-myristoyl > PEG-stearoyl after 24h incubation. Furthermore, the possibility of re-uptake of PEG-lipid into liposomal membrane was examined. The PEG-lipid solution was added to 50% FBS containing PEG-modified liposome. The amount of PEG-lipid on liposomal membrane was limited to 60% at time zero in PEG2000-DSG, while this level reached 200 % in PEG2000-DPG after 24 h. Thus, the level of residual PEG-lipid on liposomal membrane was high in PEG2000-DPG modified liposomes, suggesting it was very useful in the re-uptake of PEG-lipid by liposomal membrane. Thus, it was considered that PEG2000-DPG which had a high rate of residual PEG-lipid on liposomal membrane depended on the re-uptake of PEG-lipid to liposomal membrane.

It was expected that removement-reuptake of PEG-lipids on liposomal membrane had an influence on the effect of liposomal uptake into tumor cells. Then, it is considered that the transition of PEG-lipid into tumor cell membrane was important. PEG-lipid moved into cell membrane during incubation with tumor cells. It was speculated that PEG-lipids entered the cell membrane with time and the extent of transition was greatest in PEG2000-DPG, which agreed with the result of re-uptake of PEG-lipid by liposomal membrane.

For DOX-containing liposomes, it appeared that the antitumor activity and cell uptake were not only affected by physical properties, but also by the entrapped DOX amount, the administered lipid amount, PEG modification and anchor of PEG-lipids. Considering the prolonged circulation in the blood and the avoidance of the RES, a higher entrapped amount of DOX and any PEG-modified liposomes were shown to be useful.

2.2. Therapy of Peritoneal Dissemination

Peritoneal dissemination is a serious concern in therapy for abdominal tumors such as hepatic or gastric tumors [34]. Neither surgery nor intravenous injection of antitumor drugs prevents the dissemination [35]. For an antitumor drug to be used in therapy for peritoneal dissemination, it must: (a) be sensitive and have dose-dependent effects on the disseminated tumor; (b) not be a prodrug and have cytotoxic effects on the disseminated tumor cells; (c) show low peritoneal clearance, that is, be eliminated slowly from the abdominal cavity; and (d) not cause medicinal peritonitis [35]. However, due to the rapid elimination of drug in the abdominal cavity, the intraperitoneal injection of an antitumor drug solution has little effect on peritoneal dissemination. Chemohyperthermic peritoneal perfusion of cisplatin plus mitomycin C has proved to be an effective therapy [36,37]. However, in the case of peritoneal dissemination following excision of primary tumor, this therapy may have little efficacy [38].

Intravenous injections are commonly used in liposomal studies [39-42]. However, as therapy for solid tumor, it was tried an intraperitoneal administration of liposomes and found it to be more effective [28]. Liposomes can be transferred into the blood via the lymph node in the abdominal cavity with a reserve of liposomes maintained in the abdominal cavity. The clearance of liposomes from the abdominal cavity in detail and the efficacy of intraperitoneal liposomes on treating peritoneal dissemination were shown [43].

In small negatively charged liposomes, the difference in lipid composition did not affect the disappearance or the stability of the liposomes in the abdominal cavity. It appears that the transfer of liposome to the lymph from the abdominal cavity is not related to the lipid composition. However, there was a difference in the tissue distribution of the liposomes after their transfer to the blood from the lymph. Namely, the blood circulation in the DSPC liposome group was superior to that in the DMPC liposome group.

On the other hand, the clearance from the abdominal cavity in the DSPC liposome (particle size : 150 nm; DS(S)-Lip) group was of the same pattern as that for the DSPC liposome (600 nm; DS(M)-Lip) group. In contrast, DSPC liposome (4000 nm; DS(L)-Lip) was most abundant in the abdominal cavity among the three sizes of liposome. As the DOX levels in the heart, liver and tumor after DS(L)-Lip injection were lower than in the DS(S)-Lip group, we considered that DS(L)-Lip were disrupted slowly in the abdominal cavity and DOX was released from the liposomes. Therefore, it is clear that small liposomes are effective against solid tumor and large liposome against peritoneal dissemination. As the PEG modification of DS(S)-Lip did not influence the clearance of DOX from the abdominal cavity, the PEG modification did not affect the absorption of liposome from the lymphnodi.

However, after the absorption from the abdominal cavity, the PEG modification changed the distributions in the blood and tissues.

Furthermore, positively charged liposomes were rapidly removed and then disappeared slowly, which contrasts with the pattern for the clearance of negatively charged liposomes. Each tissue in the abdominal cavity was considered to be negatively charged, and thus positive charged DSPC liposome is electrically adsorbed by the abdominal tissues. The decrease in the zeta potential by the PEG modification reduced the adsorption of the liposomes by the abdominal tissues. For the treatment of peritoneal dissemination, it was concluded that PEG modification of positively charged liposomes is not useful. In conclusion, small and large liposomes appear to be effective against solid tumor except in the abdominal cavity, and against peritoneal dissemination in the abdominal cavity, respectively.

Many methods of preparing liposome are known and it is expected that each liposome preparation has different profiles [44]. The method of preparation probably affects physical properties, but it is not clear how the biological and physical properties of these liposomes differ. On liposomal DOX made by the Bangham method (BLDOX), pH gradient method (PLDOX) and gelation method (GLDOX), the physical properties, cell uptake of DOX and therapy for peritoneal dissemination of were examined. The intracellular level of DOX in vitro experiment increased time dependently in the BLDOX and PLDOX groups, whereas its uptake was low level in the case of GLDOX [45]. The uptake of BLDOX was two-fold of that of PLDOX. Namely, it was shown that the liposome preparation affects cell uptake of liposome in vitro. The difference in the intracellular level of DOX was considered to be affected by the amount of DOX in the lipid bilayer of the liposome, leak level of DOX from the liposome, a difference of interaction (adsorption, fusion etc.) between the liposomal lipid bilayer and tumor cell membrane, and the stability of liposomes. BLDOX contained a relatively large amount of DOX in the lipid bilayer compared to the other liposomes. It was speculated that this led to the increase in DOX uptake by the cells. In the PLDOX group, DOX was entrapped in the internal water phase of the liposome and less DOX existed in the liposomal lipid bilayer compared to in BLDOX because of the pH gradient inside and outside of the liposome. It was considered that this led to the decrease in DOX leak from liposomes. In the GLDOX group, DOX was not present in the liposomal lipid bilayer because the DOX entrapped in the internal phase of the liposome became gelated. Judging from this, GLDOX was more stable than BLDOX and PLDOX.

However, it was expected that this resulted in little uptake of DOX from GLDOX by tumor cells.

On incubation in 50% FBS, all the liposomes leaked DOX transiently for 30 min at 37°C, the order for DMPC-containing liposomes being BLDOX > PLDOX > GLDOX. In the case of BLDOX, the influence of pH change when applied to 50% FBS, and the large amount of DOX incorporated into the lipid bilayer that was expected from the zeta potentials, induced the strong leak of DOX compared to other types of liposomes. In the case of GLDOX, little DOX leaked because the internal phase of the liposomes was gelated. These results reflected the uptake of liposomal DOX by tumor cells in vitro, suggesting that the leak of DOX from liposomes was more important than endocytosis or membrane fusion of liposomes.

In the intraperitoneal administration of DOX liposomes on the survival of ascites carcinoma-bearing mice as the model of peritoneal dissemination, survival in the BLDOX group was significantly prolonged compared to that in the PLDOX and GLDOX groups [45]. In the GLDOX group, there was no effect on survival. Thus, effective drug leak from the liposomes affected the survival when administered intraperitoneally. Therefore, it was speculated that the drug was leaked from liposomes to some extent early at the local site, and prolonged exposure to DOX was important for local therapy.

In conclusion, preparation is an important factor affecting the properties of liposomes, and for local therapy like peritoneal dissemination, BLDOX is most effective because its early delivery of drug is reflected in vitro.

2.3. Mixed PEG Modified Liposomes

With PEG modification of the liposome surface, a fixed aqueous layer is formed around the liposomes by interaction between the PEG-polymer and water molecule [47], and prevents the attraction of opsonins, because, serum proteins cannot bind to the water gathered on the surface of the liposomes. As a result, PEG-modified liposomes escape trapping by the cells of the RES, have a prolonged circulation time, and accumulate in tumors by passive targeting [48-50]. However, it is difficult to insert PEG, which can be used to enlarge the fixed aqueous layer thickness (FALT), on the surface of liposomes, so effects of modification by PEG are not exhibited enough.

To increase FALT and insert ratio in liposomal membrane, mixed PEG-modified DOX liposomes was prepared, using PEG-DSG (molecular weight; 340, 500, 900, 2000). Moreover, the effects of PEG-modification of the liposome on the tissue distribution and antitumor activity of DOX in vivo, and the connection between physical character and biological properties of mixed PEG modified liposomes were clarified [51].

The FALT was increased as the PEG molecular weight increased, but the ratio of increase was reduced with PEG molecular weight (Table 1). Modeling of PEG-lipid, which modified the surface of liposomes, has shown that at least two regimes can be identified, 'mushrooms' (isolated grafts) and 'brushes' (extended chain conformations determined by the interaction between neighboring chains) [52]. This phenomenon could suggest that, because, PEG lipid with a large molecular weight constructed more complete 'mushroom' structures than that with a small molecular weight, the increase of FALT was smaller than the increase of PEG molecular weight. FALTs of PEG [500) and PEG (2000) on the basis of bond angle and bond length of polyoxyethylene chains could be tentatively calculated. Consequently, when PEG (500) and PEG (2000) formed complete 'brushes', FALTs were 4.18 and 16.72 nm. On the other hand, when they formed complete 'mushroom' structures, FALTs around liposomes were 0.73 and 2.52 nm, respectively. From these results, it was suggested that PEG-lipid with a large molecular weight constructed more complete 'mushroom' structures than that with a small molecular weight.

In contrast, the FALT of liposome modified by a mixture of PEG900 and PEG340 had a value between that of PEG(900) and that of PEG(340). On mixed modification by PEG2000 and PEG with a short polyoxyethylene chain (PEG340 or PEG500), their FALT increased in comparison with the FALT of PEG(2000). Moreover, when the surface of liposomes was modified by a mixture of PEG500 and PEG2000, the most suitable mix (PEG(2000:500=2:1)), showed a maximum FALT (Figure 1). This phenomenon was speculated to occur as follows. The mixture of PEG2000 and PEG which had a short polyoxyethylene chain increased the FALT in comparison with that of PEG(2000), because, 'mushroom' structures of PEG-lipid which has a large molecular weight became longer as a result of insertion of PEG-lipid with a short polyoxyethylene chain into the interval of a large one. At this time, if the amount of PEG-lipid, which had a small molecular weight, was too high, its FALT had a value between that of two single PEG-modified liposomes, because of the increase in area occupied by PEG-lipid, which had a small molecular weight. If the amount of PEG-lipid, which had a small molecular weight, was too low, its FALT had a similar value to that of PEG(2000), because, the effects of PEG-lipid, which had a small molecular weight, were minimal. Furthermore, it was suggested that single PEG modification by the PEG-lipid, which had a large molecular weight, couldn't display sufficient ability, whereas the mixture of PEGs, which had a long and short polyoxyethylene chain, exhibited a stronger effect on PEG-modification.

Table 1. Particle Size and FALT of PEG-DSG modified Liposomes and Plane Liposome

	Particle size (nm)	FALT (nm)
Plane liposome	128.8±2.7	0.34±0.05
PEG(340)	142.6±0.8	0.94±0.03
PEG (500)	121.3±2.0	1.00±0.01
PEG (900)	138.0±1.9	2.10±0.02
PEG (2000)	145.6±2.7	2.52±0.03
PEG (2000:500=1:2)	140.1±1.4	2.26±0.04
PEG (2000:500=1:1)	139.1±2.1	2.95±0.03
PEG (2000:500=2:1)	142.7±5.1	3.30±0.26
PEG (2000:500=4:1)	137.9±0.2	2.53±0.23

Plane Liposome: not PEG-modified liposome.
FALT: fixed aqueous layer thickness.
Particvle sizes and FALTs are expressed as means+/- S.D. ($n \geqq 3$).
PEG(340) : PEG340-DSG modified liposome.

In PEG modified liposome entrapped DOX, the DOX concentration in the plasma increased with increase of FALT, PEG-modified liposomes of large FALT being shown to maintain a high DOX level. In the livers, it was observed that DOX accumulation caused by liposomalization and avoidance from RES caused by PEG-modification. This result was supposed that the ability to avoid trapping by RES was caused by increase of FALT. While, in the tumor, the time course of the DOX concentration showed a relation between increase of FALT and maintenance of a high DOX level for a long time. Thus, PEG (2000:500 = 2:1) modified liposome entrapped DOX, with high level of FALT, was indicated to be superior antitumor effect.

PEG-alkyl lipid derivatives have different physicochemical properties depending on the molecular weight of the PEG moiety, the fatty acid length as the anchor, and the conformation of the spacer unit as the connection between the lipids and PEG. It is known that the dissociation of PEG lipid from liposomes differs according to the conformation of the anchor unit [31]. Next, mixed PEG-modified liposomes by PEG-cholesterol (PEG-CHO), which has different characteristics with the alkyl anchor as the surface material of the liposome modification, was examined. The FALT of a mixed (PEG2000-DSG and PEG2000-CHO with the same PEG-molecular weight and different anchor unit) modified liposome was 3.43 nm, more than that of the single PEG2000-DSG modified liposomes or single PEG2000-CHO modified liposomes [53]. It is thought that the increase of FALT in PEG2000-(DSG : CHO = 1:1)-LDOX is based on the following reasons: 1) only a part of the anchor units of PEG-CHO come in the liposomal membrane, the PEG chain of PEG-DSG pushes up the PEG chain of PEG-CHO, 2) PEG-CHO, where one chain is inserted into the deep position, the PEG chain of PEG-CHO pushes up the PEG chain of PEG-DSG, and PEG-DSG changes from the mushroom structure to the brush structure.

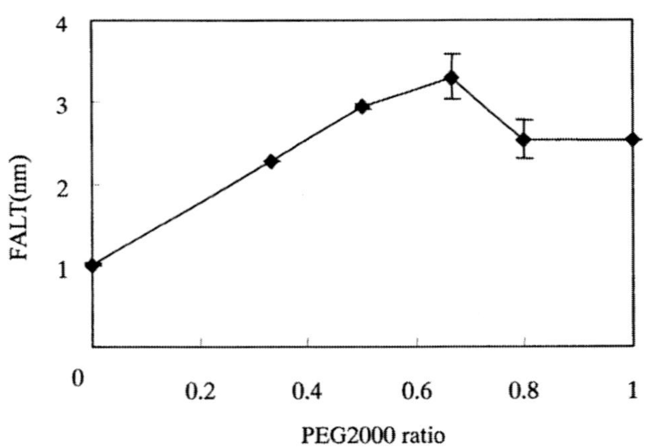

Figure 1. Effect of PEG2000 ratio on the FALT of PEG(2000:500)-DSG modified liposomes.
When PEG2000 ratio is 0, PEG500 ratio is 1. Each point represents the mean S.D. of 4 samples.

It was reported that vesicles that consist of phospholipids containing a PEG-CHO derivative have high fluidity, instability of liposomal membrane and a high affinity for cell membranes [54]. On the other hand, it is said that the PEG-CHO modification of the liposome depresses the cell uptake because the hydrophilic layer on liposomal membranes inhibits the interaction with liposomes and serum proteins or a direct connection between liposomes and cells [55]. However, PEG2000-(DSG: CHO = 1:1)-LDOX, PEG2000-CHO-

LDOX and PEG2000-DSG- LDOX had significantly increased the DOX uptake into tumor cells in the case of PLDOX after 30 min of incubation. In particular, as the cell uptake of PEG2000-CHO-LDOX was dominantly high, it was indicated that PEG-CHO has a high affinity with tumor cells. In addition, it was suggested that liposomes modified with PEG-CHO and PEG-DSG also have these characteristics. The IC_{50}, used as the index of the effect of cytotoxicity and the cell survival ratio on the tumor cells, increased in the order of PLDOX, PEG2000-DSG-LDOX, PEG2000-CHO-LDOX and PEG-2000(DSG:CHO = 1:1)-LDOX. In particular, PEG2000 -CHO-LDOX and PEG2000-(DSG:CHO = 1:1)-LDOX showed an expected cytotoxicity compared with the case of PLDOX. Namely, it was expected that mixed modified liposomes with PEG-CHO lipid cause not only the FALT but also the cell transfer and antitumor effect to be increased in vivo.

In conclusion, it was concluded that the mixed PEG-modification on the surface of liposomes gave the increase of FALT. Regarding the connection between increase of FALT and long circulation in blood, the involvement of antitumor activity of DOX of these liposomes was suggested. Moreover, by mixed PEG modifications with alkyl and cholesterol anchors, the characteristics of long-term circulation in the blood and the high cellular transfer of liposomes were formulated, their effectiveness in cancer chemotherapy is expected.

3. Combined Food Components

As to enhancing agents for antitumor drugs many detailed studies on 5-fluorouracil and cisplatin as effectors have been performed [56-58]. However, there have been few reports on increases in antitumor activity without increases in adverse reactions. The use of a modulator, which is expected to increase the antitumor agent-induced antitumor activity, increases the number of medications and thus adds to the patient’s burden. In contrast, if the intake of food or beverage as a modulator enhances the antitumor activity and exhibits no adverse reaction, it was expected that the quality of life of clinical patients will be improved. It was clarified that the combination of food components with DOX were advanced therapeutic index.

3.1. Theanine

Theanine (γ-glutamylethylamide) is a water-soluble amino acid specifically found in green tea (Camellia sinensis), comprising about 1–2% (dry weight) of green tea leaves and is one of the tastier components [59]. Regarding the effects of theanine, the inhibition of the excitation of the central nervous system by caffeine, acceleration on the synthesis of nerve growth factor, the reduction of blood pressure and acceleration of release of dopamine in brain were reported [60, 61]. Furthermore, theanine has been shown to be absorbed by a common Na^+-coupled cotransporter in the intestinal brush border membrane [62].

In the combined treatment of theanine and DOX on Ehrlich ascites carcinoma-bearing mice, DOX (2.0 mg/kg/day x 4 days) reduced the tumor growth by 25%, while theanine (10 mg/kg/day x 4 days) + DOX also decreased the tumor weight and then theanine enhanced the DOX induced inhibitory effect by 2.1-fold. The DOX concentration in the tumor in theanine combined group was significantly increased by 2.9-fold compared to DOX alone. Thus, it is demonstrated that theanine is useful as a novel biochemical modulator increasing the antitumor activity. Furthermore, in M5076 ovarian sarcoma-bearing mice, combination of theanine with DOX significantly reduced the tumor growth, whereas DOX alone slightly reduced the tumor weight, with the increase of the DOX concentration in the tumor. Namely, although M5076 sarcoma has low sensitivity to DOX, the effective antitumor activity was observed by combined theanine with DOX. M5076 sarcoma is a highly invasive and metastatic tumor and spontaneously metastasizes to the liver and lung. In a spontaneous metastasis experiment, the combined treatment of theanine with DOX was performed on M5076 tumor-bearing mice. The average of hepatic metastasis score was control group > DOX-alone group > DOX + theanine group. Theanine amplified the suppressive efficacy of DOX on hepatic metastasis. Modulators that enhance the antitumor activity of chemotherapeutic agents against primary tumors and which are also effective in inhibiting subsequent metastasis have not been reported. Therefore, theanine is indicated to be useful for enhancement of not only antitumor activity but also inhibition of metastasis induced by DOX.

Furthermore, multidrug resistance is one of the major obstacles encountered in cancer chemotherapy [63]. Some drug efflux pumps are reported to contribute to drug resistance, such as P-glycoprotein and MRPs and some agents which inhibit these pumps, such as verapamil and cyclosporin A, are utilized for reversal of drug resistance [64]. However, these drug-resistance reversal agents exhibit severe toxicity and enhance the antitumor agent-induced adverse reaction in normal tissues, so that its clinical use is probably impossible. In contrast, the combination of theanine with DOX on multidrug-resistant P388 leukemia overexpressing P-glycoprotein significantly reduced the tumor weight, while DOX alone did not change the tumor growth. A significant increase in DOX concentration in the tumor was observed by combined theanine, suggesting that theanine increases the DOX concentration not only in drug sensitive tumors but also in drug-resistant tumors.

As theanine was inhibited DOX efflux in these tumor cells, it is expected that this effect is connected with inhibition of the glutamate transporter by theanine, is glutamate derivative. However, it is difficult to believe that DOX is directly transported by the glutamate transporter. It is speculated that DOX is transported extracellularly via other transport systems and that the reduction in glutamate uptake by theanine induces a change in the amount of DOX transported.

Glutathione (GSH) is a tripeptide synthesized from cysteine, glutamate and glycine. The effect of GSH is important to the detoxification system for xenobiotics. It has been reported that the ATP-dependent glutathione S-conjugate export (GS-X) pump has something to do with the transport of antitumor agents in cell membranes [65-70]. M5076 cells were incubated with DOX and theanine or DL-buthionine sulfoximine (BSO), a specific inhibitor of γ-glutamyl-cysteine synthetase, the rate-limiting enzyme for GSH synthesis [71]. As well as BSO, theanine significantly decreased the intracellular concentration of GSH in M5076 cells. Namely, the inhibition of glutamate uptake by theanine was considered to induce a decrease in the synthesis of GSH from glutamate. Furthermore, the intracellular generation of the GS-DOX conjugate was confirmed to decrease with the theanine-induced reduction in the level of GSH. From these results, it was speculated that theanine decreased the intracellular concentration of GSH and reduced the generation of the GSH conjugate with intracellular DOX, and then the extracellular release of the GS-DOX conjugate decreased. MRPs were reported to transport the GSH conjugate ATP-dependently and to be a code for the GS-X pump [69]. In M5076 cells, the expression of MRP5, which functions in the efflux of DOX, was confirmed [72]. Namely, some of the DOX taken up by tumor cells binds to GSH and thereby generates the GS-DOX conjugate. The conjugate is released extracellularly by the MRP5/GS-X pump. On the other hand, theanine suppressed the uptake of glutamate and thereafter the biosynthesis of GSH through inhibition of glutamate transporters in M5076 cells [73]. Then, generation of the conjugate of intracellular DOX and GSH is affected and the release of the GS-DOX conjugate by tumor cells via the MRP5/GS-X pump decreases. It is considered that these phenomena suppress the decrease in the concentration of DOX in a tumor and induce the increase in the DOX induced antitumor activity caused by theanine. The glutamate transporter-mediated increase in antitumor activity caused by theanine is a novel mechanism, and it is hoped that this action will lead to the discovery of a useful cancer chemotherapy for drug-sensitive, drug-resistant and metastatic tumors.

3.2. Curucumin

Curcumin is widely used as a food coloring and flavoring agent and has wide range of pharmacological activities which include anti-inflammatory, antioxidative, and anti-angiogenic properties. Curcumin effects on cellular enzymes such as cyclooxygenase and glutathione S-transferase (GST) include a potent antioxidant capacity [74]. After an injection of DOX to M5076-bearing mice, tumor weight was not reduced. In contrast, the combination of DOX with curcumin significantly reduced the tumor weight to 56.5% ($p < 0.05$) of that of the control group [75]. However, the addition of curcumin did not increase DOX concentration in the tumors as compared to the DOX alone group.

The DOX concentration in the heart in the curcumin+DOX group was reduced to 74.2% compared with that in the DOX alone group. Furthermore, the antioxidative effect of curcumin was expected to reduce the adverse reactions of DOX. The AST and ALT levels in the serum were increased by DOX whereas the addition of curcumin had a tendency to suppress their increase. The DOX induced active oxygen species oxidize lipids in the myocardial membrane [76]. It has been reported that the reduction of glutathione peroxidase activity is particularly connected with increasing lipid peroxide (LPO) levels [77]. Curcumin with antioxidative property was able to interfere with the adverse effects of DOX attributed to the accumulation of LPO in the heart [75].

Curcumin did not suppress DOX efflux from tumor cells in vitro. These results supported the fact that the DOX concentration in the tumor did not change in vivo. Since curcumin enhanced the effect of DOX antitumor activity, it was assumed that it performed these actions via a mechanism other than membrane transport of DOX. It has been reported that curcumin caused the apoptosis of tumor cells through various pathways [78,79].

Curcumin+DOX significantly decreased cell viability by DOX. Histograms of flow cytometry indicated that the curcumin+DOX combination induced more apoptosis than DOX alone. The observation of chromatin condensation with Hoechst 33342 stain shows that treatment with curcumin and DOX induced chromatin condensation in a time dependent manner suggesting that cells were undergoing apoptosis [75].

In apoptosis pathways, one is the pathway which activates caspase-3 through activation of caspase-8 by a signal from the death receptor. Another is the pathway which activates caspase-3 through activation of caspase-9 with cytochrome c released from the mitochondria. DOX treatment of M5076 cells enhanced the activation of caspase-3 in a time- and condensation- dependent manner and the combination of curcumin suppressed activation of caspase-3 compared with DOX alone. This effect was speculated to involve the anti-oxidative effects of curcumin.

The antitumor activity of DOX is shown to be due to topoisomerase II inhibition and DNA damage through radical reactions [80,81] and apoptosis. The mechanism of apoptosis involving DOX has been due to oxidative DNA damage by DOX-induced hydrogen peroxide generation [82]. Hydrogen peroxide generated through both pathways leads to an increase in mitochondrial membrane potential and subsequent caspase-3 activation through caspase-9 activation in DOX-induced apoptosis. Thus, the antioxidative properties of curcumin were postulate to inhibit hydrogen peroxide release from DOX leading to suppressed activation of caspase-9 and -3. Curcumin suppressed the activation of caspase-9 and -8 compared to DOX alone. Viability of cells treated with curcumin and DOX was significantly lower than with DOX alone and the occurrence of apoptosis was enhanced. It was hypothesized that curcumin combined with DOX suppresses the main caspase pathway and activates the main caspase independent pathway involving apoptosis-inducing factor [83,84] and caspase-12 through endoplasmic reticulum stress [85]. Thus, curcumin is a useful modulator to enhance DOX induced antitumor activity while reducing the adverse effects.

3.3. Linalool

Humulus lupulus (hop) is used primarily for its bitter and aromatic properties in the manufacture of beer. Bitter acid, volatile oil and prenylated flavonoids are active components of hop, having anticarcinogenic effects [86], estrogenic activity [87] and anti-HIV activity [88]. The effects of myrcene, αhumulen, β-caryophyllene and linalool, which are volatile oil components in hop, on DOX permeability in tumor cells were examined.

Myrcene, a-humulen and b-caryophyllene did not have beneficial effects on DOX permeability in tumor cells. On the other hand, although linalool had no effect on DOX efflux, DOX levels in tumor cells by combination with linalool significantly increased in the DOX influx system [89]. Therefore, linalool promoted DOX influx in tumor cells and increased DOX concentration in tumor cells. Furthermore, the combination of DOX with linalool in vitro showed increased cytotoxicity compared with the effects of DOX alone. It is clear that the combination with linalool enhanced DOX cytotoxicity by an increase of DOX concentration in tumor cells.

In vivo, the combination of DOX with linalool caused a significant decrease in the tumor weight of P388 leukemia-bearing mice compared with that in the DOX alone treated group; Furthermore, it was thought that linalool increased DOX-induced antitumor activity by maintenance of the DOX concentration in the tumor. Thus, it was considered that the combination of DOX with linalool increased DOX concentration in the tumor owing to the promotion of DOX influx by linalool.

Furthermore, the effects of combination with linalool did not disappear with the change of temperature and was not affected by ATP-depleted conditions. Thus, it was suggested that the promotion of DOX influx by combined linalool does not depend on energy. In contrast, the promotion of DOX influx by linalool was suppressed by the absence of Na^+, suggesting that promotion of the DOX influx system requires the presence of Na^+. Therefore, it was suggested that the promotion of the DOX influx system by linalool that enhanced antitumor activity of DOX is related to energy independent and Na^+-dependent transporter.

The nucleoside transporter is one of the transporters related to the energy-independent and Na^+-dependent DOX permeability [90]. The nucleoside transporter family is divided into Na^+-dependent nucleoside transporter (CNT) and equilibrative nucleoside transporters (ENT). CNT is classified into CNT1, CNT2 and CNT3, while ENT is classified into ENT1, ENT2, ENT3 and ENT4 [90]. In the DOX alone treated group, the uptake rate of DOX in the presence of S-(4-nitrobenzyl)-6-thioinosine (NBMPR), as inhibitors of CNT3 and ENT1, increased in comparison with that in the absence of NBMPR group. ENT is bi-directional, and acts mainly as efflux systems under physiological condition. So, the increased uptake in the presence of NBMPR could be due to inhibition of DOX efflux via ENT1. The promoting effect of linalool on DOX uptake was inhibited by the presence of NBMPR, suggesting that the promoted

DOX influx is related to CNT3. In terms of the effects of phlorizin, as an inhibitor of CNT3, on the uptake of DOX, the promoting effect of linalool on DOX influx was inhibited. Thus, it is considered that the increase of linalool induced DOX influx was due to promotion of DOX influx through CNT3 by linalool. CNT3 is not found in the heart as normal tissue [90], and thus linalool did not increase DOX concentration in the heart.

In conclusion, it is considered that linalool promoted DOX influx in tumor cells because of its action on DOX transport through CNT3, which increased DOX concentration in tumor cells and then enhanced the antitumor activity of DOX with reduced adverse reactions of DOX.

3.4. Other Compounds

Anserine (a dipeptide contained in fowl and migratory fish) was increased DOX induced antitumor activity with the elevation of DOX concentration in the tumor [91]. Anserine considered to take into tumor cells via a dipeptide transporter, and it resulted in an increase of the DOX influx in tumor cells. Taurine (a major amino acid in fish and meat) and cucurbitacin E and I (a bitter tasting component of squash fruit) co-treatment were confirmed to increase DOX induced antitumor activity without an increase in adverse reactions by DOX, too [92-94]. Namely, it was clarified that some foods and their components were useful as a modulator to enhance the therapeutic index of cancer patients and improve quality of life.

CONCLUSION

Advanced therapies of doxorubicin by carrier of drug delivery system or combined food components have been clarified.

In DOX liposomalization, it appeared that the antitumor activity and cell uptake were not only affected by physical properties, but also by the entrapped DOX amount, the administered lipid amount, PEG modification and anchor of PEG-lipids. Considering the prolonged circulation in the blood and the avoidance of the RES, a higher entrapped amount of DOX and PEG-modified liposomes were shown to be useful. Furthermore, preparation method is an important factor affecting the properties of liposomes, and for local therapy like peritoneal dissemination, DOX contained liposome by Bangham method is most effective because its early delivery of drug is reflected in vitro.

The FALT and antitumor activity with blood circulation and the increase of DOX concentration in the tumor increased in mixed PEG-modified DOX containing liposomes with long polyoxyethylene chains and short polyoxyethylene chains, more than single PEG modified DOX containing liposomes. Mixed PEG modified liposome with PEG-DSG and PEG-CHO led to increase in FALT and effectively increase cytotoxicity.

On the other hand, DOX of combination with food components have been useful. Theanine increased the DOX concentration in a tumor in vivo through inhibition of the glutamate transporter via the GS-X pump. The glutamate transporter-mediated increase in antitumor activity caused by theanine is a novel mechanism, and it is expected that this action will lead to the discovery of useful cancer chemotherapy for drug-sensitive, drug-resistant and metastatic tumors.

Curcumin is a useful modulator to enhance DOX induced antitumor activity while reducing the adverse effects by suppressing lipid peroxidation in normal tissue. The mechanism by which curcumin enhances DOX antitumor activity is considered to involve main caspase-independent cell death. Furthermore, useful food elements such as linalool, anserine and taurine will be hoped to bring about an improvement in clinical cancer therapy and QOL of patients who take advantage of the benefits of these substances.

Advanced therapies of DOX by liposomalization of DOX or combined food components with DOX was expected to contribute to clinical cancer chemotherapy in the future.

REFERENCES

[1] D.A. Gewirtz, A critical evaluation of the mechanism of action proposed for the antitumor effects of the anthracycline antibiotics adriamycin and daunorubicin. *Biochem. Pharmacol.,* 57, 727-741 (1999).

[2] K.S. Carter, The clinical evaluation of analogs-III. Anthracyclines. *Cancer Chemother. Pharmacol.,* 4, 5-10 (1980).

[3] E. DelaFlor-Weiss, B. Uziely, F.M. Muggia, Protracted drug infusions in cancer treatment: an appraisal of 5-fluorouracil, doxorubicin, and platinums. *Ann. Oncol.,* 4, 723-733 (1993).

[4] C.E. Myers, W.P. McGuire, R.H. Liss, I. Ifrim, K. Grotzinger, R.C. Young, Adriamycin: the role of lipid peroxidation in cardiac toxicity and tumor response. *Science,* 197, 165-167 (1977).

[5] J. Goodman, P. Hochstein, Generation of free radicals and lipid peroxidation by redox cycling of adriamycin and daunomycin. *Biochem. Biophys. Res. Commun.*, 77, 797-803 (1977).

[6] X. Luo, Y. Evrovsky, D. Cole, J. Trines, L.N. Benson, D.C. Lehotay, Doxorubicin-induced acute changes in cytotoxic aldehydes, antioxidant status and cardiac function in the rat. *Biochim. Biophys. Acta,* 1360, 45-52 (1997).

[7] E. L. Gervasoni, Z.S. Fields, S. Krishn, A.M. Baker, M. Rosado, K. Thuraisamy, A.A. Hindenberg, N.R. Taub, N.R., Subcellular distribution of daunorubicin in P-glycoprotein -positive and -negative drug-resistant cell line using laser-assisted confocal microscopy. *Cancer Res.,* 51, 4955-4963 (1991).

[8] S. Ishikawa, D.C. Wright, H. Ishizuka, GS-X pump is functionally overexpressed in cis-diamminedichloroplatinum (II) resistant human leukemia HL-60 cells and downregulated by cell differentiation. *J. Biol. Chem.,* 269, 29085-29093 (1994).

[9] M. Kool, M. Haas, G.L. Scheffer, R.J. Scheper, M.J.T. Van Eijk, J.A. Juijin, F. Baas, P. Borst, Analysis of expression of cMOAT(MRP2), MRP3, MRP4 and MRP5, homologues of the multidrug resistance-associated protein gene (MRP1), in human cancer cell lines. *Cancer Res.,* 57, 3537-3547 (1997).

[10] W. Priebe, M. Krawczyk, T.M. Kuo, Y. Yamane, N. Savaraj, T. Ishikawa, Doxorubicin- and daunorubicin–glutathione conjugates, but not unconjugated drugs, competitively inhibit leukotriene C4 transport mediated by MRP/GS-X pump. *Biochem. Biophys. Res. Commun.*, 247, 859-863 (1998).

[11] P. Borst, R. Evers, M. Kool, J. Wijnholds, The multidrug resistance protein family. *Biochim. Biophys. Acta,* 1461, 347-357 (1999).

[12] T. Sumizawa, Z.S. Chen, Y. Chuman, K. Seto, T. Furusawa, M. Haraguchi, A. Tani, N. Shudo, S. Akiyama, Reversal of multidrug resistant-associated proteinmediated drug resistance by the pyridine analog PAK-104P. *Mol. Pharmacol.,* 51, 399-405 (1977).

[13] T. Tsuruo, H. Iida, M. Nojiri, S. Tsukagoshi, Y. Sakurai, Circumvention of vincristine and adriamycin resistance in vitro and in vivo by calcium influx blocker. *Cancer Res.,* 43, 2905-2910 (1983).

[14] K. Yusa, T. Tsuruo, Reversal mechanism of multidrug resistance by verapamil: direct binding of verapamil to P-glycoprotein on specific sites and transport of verapamil outward across the plasma membrane of K562/ADM cells. *Cancer Res.,* 46, 5002-5006 (1989).

[15] S. Leonce, A. Pierre, M. Anstett, V. Perez, A. Genton, J.P. Bizzari, G. Atassi, Effects of a new triazinoaminopiperidine derivative on adriamycin accumulation and retention in cells displaying P-glycoprotein-mediated multidrug resistance. *Biochem. Pharmacol.,* 44, 1707-1715 (1992).

[16] A.F. Castro, G.A. Altenberg, Inhibition of the drug transport by genisteine in multidrug-resistant cells expressing P-glycoprotein. *Biochem. Pharmacol.,* 53, 89-93 (1997).

[17] F. Bichat, G. Solis-Recebdez, M.G. Poullatin, M.F. Poupon, D. Khayat, G. Bastian, S9788 modulation of P-glycoprotein and multidrug-related protein-mediated multidrug resistance by servier 9788 in doxorubicin-resistant MCF7 cells. *Biochem. Pharmacol.,* 56, 497-502 (1998).

[18] N. Kusunoki, K. Takara, Y. Tanigawa, A. Yamaguchi, K. Ueda, F. Komada, Y. Ku, Y. Kuroda, Y. Saitoh, K. Okumura, Inhibitory effects of cyclosporine derivative, SDZ PSC 833, on transport of doxorubicin and vinblastine via P-glycoprotein. *Jpn. J. Cancer Res.,* 89, 1220-1228 (1998).

[19] M.D. Bruin, K. Miyake, T. Litman, R. Robey, S.E. Bates, Reversal of resistance by GF120918 in cell lines expressing the ABC half-transporter, MXR. *Cancer Lett.,* 146, 117-126 (1999).

[20] R.S. Benjamin, C.E. Riggs, N.R. Bauchur, Plasma pharmacokinetics of Adriamycin and its metabolite in humans with normal hepatic and renal function. *Cancer Res.,* 37, 1416-1420(1977).

[21] S. Shinozawa, T. Oda, Determination of Adriamycin (doxorubicin) and related fluorescent compound in rat lymph and gall by high-performance liquid chromatography. *J. Chromatogr.* 212, 323-330 (1981).

[22] A.M.B. Bots, W.J. Oort, Q.G.C.M. Hoesel, Analysis of Adriamycin and adriamycinol in micro volumes of rat plasma. *J. Chromatogr.* 272, 421-427 (1983).

[23] S. Eksborg, U. Stendahl, U. Lonroth, Comparative pharmacokinetic study of Adriamycin and 4'-epi-adriamycin after their simultaneous intravenous administration. *Eur. J. Clin. Pharmacol.,* 30, 629-631 (1986).

[24] D.W. Yesair, E. Schwrtzbach, D. Shuk, E. Deine, M.A. Asbell, Comparative pharmacokinetics of daunomycin and Adriamycin in several animal species. *Cancer Res.,* 32, 1177-1183 (1972).

[25] R.A. Minow, R.S. Benjamin, J.A. Gottlied, Adriamycin cardiomyopathy: an overview with determination of risk factors. *Cancer Chemother. Rep*., 6, 195-201 (1975).

[26] D.D. Von Hoff, M.W. Layard, P. Basa, H.L. Davis, A.L. Von Hoff, M. Rozencweig, F.W. Muggia. Risk factors for doxorubicin-induced congestive heart failure, *Ann. Intern. Med.,* 91, 710-717 (1979).

[27] P.S. Gill, B.M. Espina, F. Muggia, S. Cabriales, A. Tulpule, J.A. Esplin, H.A. Liebman, E. Forssen, M.E. Ross, M. Levine. Phase I/II clinical and pharmacokinetic evaluation of liposomal daunorubicin. *J. Clin. Oncol.,* 13, 996-1003 (1995).

[28] Y. Sadzuka, S. Nakai, A. Miyagishima, Y. Nozawa, S. Hirota, Effects of administrated route on tissue distribution and antitumor activity of polyethyleneglycol-coated liposomes containing adriamycin. *Cancer Lett.,* 111, 77-86 (1997).

[29] Y. Sadzuka, S. Nakai, A. Miyagishima, Y. Nozawa, S. Hirota, The effects of dose on the distribution of adriamycin encapsulated in polyethyleneglycol-coated liposomes. *J. Drug Targeting,* 3, 31-37 (1995).

[30] A.D. Bangham, M.M.Standish, J.C. Watlcin, Diffusion of univalent ion across the lamellae of swollen phospholipids. *J. Mol. Biol.,* 13, 238-252 (1965).

[31] Y. Sadzuka, S. Hirota, Does the amount of an antitumor agent entrapped in liposomes influence its tissue distribution and cell uptake? *Cancer Lett.,* 131, 163-170 (1998).

[32] R. Hong, C. Hung, Y. Tseng, V. Pang, S. Chen, J. Liu, F. Chang, Direct comparison of liposomal doxorubicin with or without polyethyleneglycol coating in C-26 tumor-bearing mice is surface coating with polyethyleneglycol beneficial? *Clin. Cancer Res.,* 5, 3645-3652 (1999).

[33] Y. Sadzuka, K. Kishi, S. Hirota, T. Sonobe. Effect of polyethyleneglycol (PEG) chain on cell uptake of PEG-modified liposome. *J. Liposome Res.,* 13, 157-172 (2003).

[34] Y. Yonemura, T. Fujimura, Hyperthermo–chemotherapy and peritoneal carcinomatosis. J. *Clin. Exp. Med.,* 185, 362-365 (1998).

[35] S. Tsujitani, N. Kaibara, Intraperitoneal administration of hypotonic cisplatin solution for peritoneal dissemination of gastric cancer. *J. Clin. Exp. Med.,* 185, 357-361 (1998).

[36] S. Koga, R. Hamazoe, M. Maeta, Prophylactic therapy for peritoneal recurrence of gastric cancer by continuous hyperthermic peritoneal perfusion with mitomycin C. *Cancer,* 61, 232-237 (1988).

[37] Y. Fujimura, Y. Yonemura, K. Muraoka, Continuous hyperthermic peritoneal perfusion for the prevention of peritoneal recurrence of gastric cancer: randomized controlled study. *World J. Surg.,* 18, 150-155 (1994).

[38] N. Kaibara, M. Maeta, R. Hamazoe, Hyperthermia adjunct to surgery in the treatment of scirrhous carcinoma of the stomach. *Jpn. J. Cancer Chemother.,* 15, 1269-1272 (1988).

[39] A.L. Klibanov, K. Maruyama, V.P. Torchilin, Amphipathic polyethyleneglycols effectively prolong the circulation time of liposomes. *FEBS Lett.,* 267, 235-237 (1990).

[40] T.M. Allen, C. Hansen, F. Martin, Liposomes containing synthetic lipid derivatives of polyethylene glycol show prolonged circulation half-lives in vivo. *Biochim. Biophys. Acta,* 1066, 29-36 (1991).

[41] A.L. Klibanov, K. Maruyama, A.M. Beckerleg, A.M., Activity of amphipathic poly(ethyleneglycol) 5000 to prolong the circulation time of liposomes depends on the liposome size and its unfavorable for immunoliposome binding to target. *Biochim. Biophys. Acta,* 1062, 142-148 (1991).

[42] A. Mori, A.L. Klibanov, V.P. Torchilin, Influence of the ateric barrier activity of amphipathic poly(ethyleneglycol) and ganglioside GM1 on the circulation time of liposomes and on the target binding of immunoliposomes in vivo. *FEBS Lett.,* 284, 263-266 (1991).

[43] Y. Sadzuka, S. Hirota, T. Sonobe, Intraperitoneal administration of doxorubicin encapsulating liposomes against peritoneal dissemination. *Toxicol. Lett.,* 116, 51-59 (2000).

[44] N. Oku, *Preparation and Experimentation of Liposome*. Hirokawa Publishing Co., Tokyo, pp. 43-63 (1994).

[45] Y. Sadzuka, R. Hirama, T. Sonobe, Effect of intraperitoneal administration of liposomes and methods of preparing liposomes for local therapy. *Toxicol. Lett.,* 126, 83-90 (2000).

[46] C.D. Stubbs, K. Kinoshita Jr., F. Munkonge, P.J. Quinn, A. Ikegami, A., The dynamics of lipid motion in sarcoplasmic reticulum membranes determined by steadystate and time-resolved fluorescence measurements on 1,6-diphenyl-1,3,5-hexatriene and related molecules. *Biochem. Biophys. Acta,* 775, 374-380 (1984).

[47] K. Shimada, A. Miyagishima, Y. Sadzuka, Y. Nozawa, Y. Mochizuki, H. Ohshima, S. Hirota, Detemination of the thickness of the fixed aqueous layer around the polyethyleneglycol-coated liposomes. *J. Drug Targeting,* 3, 283-289 (1995).

[48] N.Z. Wu, D. Da, T.L. Rudoll, D. Needham, A.R. Whorton, W. Dewhist, Increased microvascular permeability contributes to preferential accumulation of stealth liposomes in tumor tissue. *Cancer Res.,* 53, 3765-3770 (1993).

[49] S. Schmitz, T.M. Allen, K. Jimbow, Polyethyleneglycol-mediated delivery of liposome -entrapped pigment into fibroblasts: experimental pigment cells as models for mutator phenotypes. *Cancer Res.,* 52, 6638-6645 (1992).

[50] D. Papafadjopoulos, T.M. Allen, A. Gabizon, E. Mayhew, K.S. Matthay, K. Huang, K.D. Lee, M.C. Woodle, D.D. Lasic, C. Redemann, F.J. Martin, Sterically stabilized liposomes: improvements in pharmacokinetics and antitumor therapeutic efficacy. *Proc. Natl. Acad. Sci.* USA, 88, 11460-11464 (1991).

[51] Y. Sadzuka, A. Nakade, R. Hirama, A. Miyagishima, Y. Nozawa, S. HIrota, T. Sonobe, Effect of mixed polyethyleneglycol modification on fixed aqueous layer thickness and antitumor activity of doxorubicin containing liposome. *Int. J. Pharm.,* 238, 171-180 (2002).

[52] D. Needham, N. Stoicheva, D.V. Zhelev, Exchange of monooleoylphosphtidylcholine as monomer and micelle with membranes containing poly(ethylene glycol)–lipid. *Biophys. J.,* 73, 2615-2629 (1997).

[53] Y. Sadzuka, I. Sugiyama, T. Tsuruda, T. Sonobe, Characterization and cytotoxicity of mixed polyethyleneglycol modified liposomes containing doxorubicin. *Int. J. Pharm.,* 312, 83-89 (2006).

[54] C. Carrion, J.C. Domingo, M.A. Madariaga, Preparation of long circulation immunoliposomes using PEG-cholesterol conjugates: effect of the spacer arm between PEG and cholesterol on liposomal characteristics. *Chem. Phys. Lipids,* 113, 97-110 (2001).

[55] S. Beugin-Deroo, M. Ollivon, S. Lesieur, Bilayer stability and impermeability of nonionic surfactant vesicles sterically stabilized by PEG cholesterol conjugates. *J. Colloid Interf. Sci.,* 202, 324-333 (1998).

[56] O.F. Hidalgo, F. Gonzalez, A. Gil, W. Campbell, E. Barrajon, A.J. Lacave, 120 Hours simultaneous infusion of cisplatin and fluorouracil in metastatic breast cancer. *Am. J. Clin. Oncol.,* 12, 397-401 (1989).

[57] Y. Ichinose, N. Takanashi, T. Yano, A phase III trial of oral tegafur and uracil plus cisplatin in patients with inoperable nonsmall cell lung cancer. *Cancer,* 75, 2677-2680 (1995).

[58] Y. Kubota, M. Hosaka, S. Fukushima, I. Kondo, Prophylactic oral UFT therapy for superficial bladder cancer. *Cancer,* 71, 1842-1845 (1993).

[59] H.N. Graham, Green tea composition, consumption, and polyphenol chemistry. *Prev. Med.,* 21, 334-350 (1992).

[60] T. Unno, Y. Suzuki, T. Kakuda, T. Hayakawa, H. Tsuge, Metabolism of theanine, γ-glutamylethylamide, in rats. *J. Agric. Food Chem.,* 47, 1593-1596 (1999).

[61] H. Yokogoshi, M. Kobayashi, M. Mochizuki, T. Terashima, Effect of theanine, γ-glutamylethylamide, on brain monoamines and striatal dopamine release in conscious rats. *Neurochem. Res.,* 25, 667-673 (1998).

[62] S. Kitaoka, H. Hayashi, H. Yokogoshi, Y. Suzuki, Transmural potential changes associated with the in vitro absorption of theanine in the guinea pig intestine. *Biosci. Biotech. Biochem.,* 60, 1768-1771 (1996).

[63] S.M. Simon, M. Schindlert, Cell biological mechanisms of multidrug resistance in tumors. *Proc. Natl. Acad. Sci. USA* 91, 3497–3504 (1994).

[64] Y. Kang, P.R. Perry, Effect of gamma-interferon on P-glycoprotein expression and function and on verapamil modulation of doxorubicin resistance. *Cancer Res.* 54, 2952–2958 (1994).

[65] T. Ishikawa, The ATP-dependent glutathione S-conjugate export pump. *Trends Biochem. Sci.,* 17, 463–468 (1992).

[66] T. Ishikawa, C.D. Wright, H. Ishizuka, GS-X pump is functionally overexpressed in cis-diamminedichloro-platinum(II)-resistant human leukemia HL-60 cells and down regulated by cell differentiation. *J. Biol. Chem.,* 269, 29085–29093 (1994).

[67] T. Ishikawa, Z. Li, Y. Lu, P.A. Rea, The GS-X pump in plant, yeast, and animal cells: structure, function, and gene expression. *Biosci. Rep.,* 17, 189–207 (1997).

[68] T. Ishikawa, The GS-X pump family: ATP dependent multispecific organic anion transporters. *Protein, Nucleic Acid, Enzyme,* 42, 1285–1294 (1997).

[69] W. Priebe, M. Krawczyk, M.T. Kuo, Y. Yamane, N. Savaraj, T. Ishikawa, Doxorubicin- and daunorubicin glutathione conjugates, but not unconjugated drugs, competitively inhibit leukotriene C4 transport mediated by MRP/GS-X pump. *Biochem. Biophys. Res. Commun.,* 247, 859–863 (1998).

[70] K. Zhang, E.B. Yang, K.P. Wong, P. Mack, GSH, GSH-related enzymes and GS-X pump in relation to sensitivity of human tumor cell lines to chlorambucil and adriamycin. *Int. J. Oncol.,* 14, 861–867 (1999).

[71] O.W. Griffith, A. Meister, Potent and specific inhibition of glutathione synthesis by buthionine sulfoximine (S-n-butyl homocysteine sulfoximine). *J. Biol. Chem.,* 254, 7558–7560 (1979).

[72] T. Sugiyama, Y. Sadzuka, K. Tanaka, T. Sonobe, Inhibition of glutamate transporter by theanine enhances the therapeutic efficacy of doxorubicin. *Toxicol. Lett.,* 121, 89-96 (2001).

[73] Y. Sadzuka, T. Sugiyama, T. Suzuki, T. Sonobe, Enhancement of the activity of doxorubicin by inhibition of glutamate transporter. *Toxicol. Lett.,* 123, 159-167 (2001).

[74] R.A. Sharma, A.J. Gescher, W.P. Steward, Curcumin: the story so far. *Eur. J. Cancer,* 41, 1955-1968 (2005).

[75] Y. Sadzuka, M. Nagamine, T. Toyooka, Y. Ibuki, T. Sonobe, Beneficial effects of curcumin on antitumor activity and adverse reactions of doxorubicin, *Int. J. Pharm.,* 432, 42-49 (2012).

[76] Y. Sazuka, K. Yoshikawa, H. Tanizawa, Y. Takino, Effect of doxorubicin on lipid peroxide levels in tissues of mice. *Jpn. J. Cancer Res.,* 78, 1281-1286 (1987).

[77] Y. Sazuka, H. Tanizawa, Y. Takino, Effect of adriamycin on the activities of superoxide dismutase, glutathione peroxidase and catalase in tissues of mice. *Jpn. J. Cancer Res.,* 80, 89-94 (1989).

[78] G.R. Pillai, A.S. Srivastava, T.I. Hassanein, D.P. Chauhan, E. Carrier, Induction of apoptosis in human lung cancer cells by curcumin. *Cancer Lett.,* 208, 163-170 (2004).

[79] S. Mishra, N. Kapoor, A.M. Ali, B.V. Pardhasaradhi, A.L. Kumari, A. Khar, K. Misra, Differential apoptotic and redox regulatory activities of curcumin and its derivatives. *Free Radic. Biol. Med.,* 38, 1353-1360 (2005).

[80] Y. Sadzuka, M. Nagamine, T. Toyooka, Y. Ibuki, T. Sonobe, Beneficial effects of curcumin on antitumor activity and adverse reactions of doxorubicin, *Int. J. Pharm.,* 432, 42-49 (2012).

[81] K. Jung, R. Reszka, Mitochondria as subcellular targets for clinically useful anthracyclines. *Adv. Drug Deliv. Rev.,* 49, 87–105 (2001).

[82] L.H. Hurley, DNA and its associated processes as targets for cancer therapy. *Nat. Rev. Cancer,* 2, 188–200 (2002).

[83] H. Mizutani, S. Tada-Oikawa, Y. Hiraku, M. Kojima, S. Kawanishi, Mechanism of apoptosis induced by doxorubicin through the generation of hydrogen peroxide. *Life Sci.,* 76, 1439-1453 (2005).

[84] C. Candé, I. Cohen, E. Daugas, L. Ravagnan,N. Larochette, N. Zamzami, G. Kroemer, Apoptosis-inducing factor (AIF): a novel caspase-independent death effector released from mitochondria. *Biochimie,* 84, 215-222 (2002).

[85] T. Arimura, A. Kojima-Yuasa, M. Suzuki, D.O. Kennedy, I. Matsui-Yuasa., Caspase-independent apoptosis induced by evening primrose extract in Ehrlich ascites tumor cells. *Cancer Lett.,* 201, 9-16 (2003).

[86] J. Li, B. Lee, A.S. Lee, Endoplasmic reticulum stress-induced apoptosis. Multiple pathways and activation of p53-up-regulated modulator of apoptosis (PUMA) and NOXA by p53. *J. Biol. Chem.,* 281, 7260-7270 (2006).

[87] H. Nozawa, W. Nakao, F. Zhao, K. Kondo, Dietary supplement of isohumulones inhibits the formation of aberrant crypt foci with a concomitant decrease in prostaglandin E2 level in rat colon. *Mol. Nutr. Food Res.,* 49, 772-778 (2005).

[88] N.G. Coldham, M.J. Sauer, Identification, quantitation and biological activity of phytoestrogens in a dietary supplement for breast enhancement. *Food Chem. Toxicol.,* 39, 1211-1224 (2001).

[89] Q. Wang, Z.H. Ding, J.K. Liu, Y.T. Zheng, Xanthohumol, a novel anti-HIV-1 agent purified from hops Humulus lupulus. *Antiviral Res.,* 64, 189-194 (2004).

[90] M. Miyashita, Y. Sadzuka, Effect of linalool as a component of Humulus lupulus on doxorubicin-induced antitumor activity. *Food Chem. Toxicol.,* 53, 174-179 (2013).

[91] J.H. Gray, R.P. Owen, K.M. Giacomini, The concentrative nucleoside transporter family, SLC28. *Pflugers Arch.,* 447, 728-734 (2004).

[92] Y. Sadzuka, T. Sonobe, Anserine induced advantage effects on the antitumor activity of doxorubicin. *Food Chem. Toxicol.,* 45, 985-989 (2007).

[93] Y. Sadzuka, M. Matuura, T. Sonobe, The effect of taurine, a novel biochemical modulator, on the antitumor activity of doxorubicin. *Biol. Pharm. Bull.,* 32, 1584-1587 (2009).

[94] Y. Sadzuka, H. Hatakeyama, T. Sonobe, Enhancement of doxorubicin concentration in the M5076 ovarian sarcoma cells by cucurbitacin E co-treatment. *Int. J. Pharm.,* 383, 186-191 (2010).

[95] Y. Sadzuka, S. Fujiki, S. Itai, Enhancement of doxorubicin-induced antitumor activity and reduction of adverse reactions by *cucurbitacin I. Food Res. Int.,* 47, 64-69 (2012).

In: Doxorubicin
Editor: Melinda Pache
ISBN: 978-1-63117-233-5

Chapter 5

PREVENTION AND MANAGEMENT OF CARDIOTOXICITY, NAUSEA AND VOMITING IN DOXORUBICIN-TREATED BREAST CANCER PATIENTS

Snezana K. Bjelogrlic[1], Snezana Susnjar[2] and Nebojsa Ninkovic[3]

[1]Department of Experimental Oncology, National Cancer Research Center, Belgrade, Serbia

[2]Department of Medical Oncology, National Cancer Research Center, Belgrade, Serbia

[3]Coronary Care Unit, University Hospital Bezanijska Kosa, Belgrade, Serbia

ABSTRACT

Despite the constant development of new drugs and biologic agents that have been introduced into cancer therapeutics, for decades doxorubicin (Doxo) remains the frontline drug against cancers, sarcomas, and hematological malignancies. Unfortunately, doxorubicin is not specifically targeting tumor agent and it also affects healthy tissues.

According to World Health Organization, breast cancer (BC) is the most frequent solid tumor in women worldwide, affecting more than a million subjects every year. Although it is well recognized that there are several molecular BC subtypes responsive to specific antineoplastic therapy, which is the step forward to individualized treatment, chemotherapy, including Doxo, is still indicated in the majority of BC patients. BC is a curable disease if it is diagnosed in early stages and afterwards treated with adjuvant full dose-intensity Doxo chemotherapy. This gives special importance to the strategy for prevention and management of its side effects. Successful use of Doxo is interrupted with a wide spectrum of toxicities, including acute nausea and vomiting, cardiotoxicity, myelosuppression, hepatotoxicity, gastrointestinal problems, renal toxicity and brain toxicity as usually seen in clinical practice. The main reason for Doxo withdrawal in BC patients is chemotherapy–induced emesis, while the major concern in the decision making process about continuation of treatment is Doxo–induced cardiotoxicity. Doxo is never applied as a single drug to BC patients, but most frequently in combination with cyclophosphamide (AC regimen). The AC regimen is recently recognized as highly-emetogenic, especially in younger women, despite the fact that each drug in this combination is of moderate emetogenic potential. Because of that the proper antiemetic prophylaxis is mandatory, including the use of NK1 and 5HT3 inhibitors, besides corticosteroids. Because heart damage is the greatest risk of Doxo-induced toxicity its administration must be dose-limited. If a lifetime accumulation of Doxo exceeds the recommended 450 mg/m^2, 50% of patients would experience measurable functional impairment, while more than 26% of them would develop congestive heart failure. Several approaches have been tested with the attempt to lower the risk of cardiac damage, such as Doxo administration as 96h infusion, liposomal Doxo delivery system, and various cardioprotective agents.

In this review we will summarize evidence and facts on prevention and management of Doxo cardiotoxicity, nausea and vomiting, based on literature data and our experience.

Introduction

Since its introduction into the protocols for treatment of metastatic breast cancer (MBC), the efficacy and tolerability of anthracyclines, and among them particularly doxorubicin (Doxo), have been widely investigated. Ultimately, this resulted in the extension of their indication for treatment of early BC (EBC) with curative intent.

The first meta-analysis showing significant improvement in both disease-free survival (DFS) and overall survival (OS) between women with EBC achieved with anthracycline-containing polychemotherapy over standard CMF (cyclophosphamide, methotrexat, 5-fluorouracil) therapy was published 15 years ago [1]. Anthracycline regimens usually included Doxo or epirubicine combined with 5-fluorouracil and cyclophosphamide (e.g., FAC or FEC). Randomized trials with direct comparisons of these two regimens with CMF chemotherapy showed significant improvement in reducing the 5-year risk of disease relapse (2p=0.006) and mortality (2p=0.02).

Another meta-analysis showed that 6 cycles of FAC/FEC therapy had reduced the annual breast cancer (BC) death rate by 38% and 20% for patients aged ≤ 50 years and 50 - 69 years, respectively [2]. The main finding from this analysis was that generally the magnitude of the risk of disease relapse reduction achieved by chemotherapy in comparison with no therapy did not change from 5 to 15 years of follow-up, while the magnitude of risk of BC death reduction was constantly increasing from the diagnosis up to 15 years of follow-up (for women aged ≤ 50 years 5-year and 15-year difference in death rates were 4.7% and 10%, respectively). In the accompanying editorial [3] the authors concluded that this widening of BC survival curves was probably caused by the chemotherapy-achieved prevention of relapses during the first 5 years.

Recently published meta-analysis including more than 100,000 women with EBC treated within 123 randomized trials [4] showed that 4 cycles of AC (Doxo 60 mg/m^2, cyclophosphamide 600 mg/m^2 per cycle) are equivalent to 6 cycles of classical CMF. However, 6 cycles of CAF/CEF cycles with higher cumulative doses of anthracyclines (360 mg Doxo/720 mg Epirubicine) were superior to CMF in reducing the 5-year BC recurrence (RR 0.77, 2p=0.0003) and mortality (RR 0.78, 2p=0.0004) [5-7].

This report [4] also included the comparison of adding taxanes (paclitaxel/docetaxel) to anthracycline-containing regimens with the same (unconfounding analysis) or a higher dose of non-taxane therapy in patients predominantly with node-positive BC. In the former trials combined therapy was usually compared to 4 cycles of AC and follow up did not exceed 8 years. Absolute gain of 4.6% (34.8% vs. 30.2%, 2p<0.00001) in survival w/o disease recurrence was achieved by adding taxane therapy. Significant absolute gain of 2.8% in reducing BC mortality (23.9% vs. 21.1%, 2p=0.0005) and 3.2% in reducing overall mortality (26.7% vs. 23.5%, 2p=0.0002) were also achieved by adding taxanes. Contrary to these results, when the control arm consisted of the same or higher doses of anthracyclines, the corresponding 5-year gains by adding taxanes were as follows: 2.9% (22% vs. 19.2%, 2p<0.00001) for DFS, 1.4% (11.5% vs. 10.1%, 2p=0.001) for BC mortality and 1.2% (12.4% vs. 11.2%, 2p=0.008) for overall mortality. Proportional risk reduction was largely independent of age, estrogen receptor (ER) status, tumor size and differentiation, and nodal status. However, there is a substantial body of evidence that adding adjuvant chemotherapy to endocrine therapy does not improve disease outcome in ER-positive/HER2-negative BC patients with low proliferative index which are surrogate markers for luminal A–like tumors [8, 9] and, more specifically, in tumors with low recurrence score (RS) even in the node positive group [10]. Not all studies confirmed this association [11], nor was ER status found to be of predictive value for response to adjuvant chemotherapy in recent EBCTCG analysis [4], but authors clearly stated that there is no information about tumor gene expression markers or quantitative immunohistochemistry that might predict risk, chemosensitivity or both. In short, meta-analysis is not an appropriate tool for investigating subset events [12].

It was proved earlier that the escalation of the Doxo dose per cycle (60 vs. 75 vs. 90 mg/m^2), thus increasing the cumulative dose per protocol, did not improve the disease outcome [13]. However, dose dense strategy did improve the disease outcome by giving the same dose of Doxo and paclitaxel every 2 weeks with GCSF support instead every 3 weeks [14].

Doxo-containing regimens are the constituents of the majority of adjuvant protocols designed for HER2-positive BC patents to be given sequentially with HER2-directed therapy. Although there is an evidence from one phase III study that anthracycline chemotherapy could be omitted from adjuvant protocol without compromising efficacy [15], anthracyclines still remain the main part of adjuvant chemotherapy regimens in these patients.

The first results of pivotal adjuvant studies in HER2–positive EBC showed an almost halved risk reduction of disease relapse and BC mortality if trastuzumab was added to anthracyclines and taxanes chemotherapy and this has not changed over time with longer follow-up [16, 17].

Recent Cochraine analysis included almost 12,000 women with early and locally advanced HER2+ BC treated within randomized clinical trials, which compared efficacy and safety of trastuzumab alone or in combination with chemotherapy or chemotherapy alone. Analysis showed that trastuzumab containing regiments significantly improves DFS (HR 0.66; 95% CI 0.57 to 0.77, $P < 0.00001$) and OS HR 0.60; 95% CI 0.50 to 0.71, $P < 0.00001$). This improvement is achieved with the cost of a higher cardiotoxicity rate: for congestive heart failure (CHF) RR 5.11; 90% CI 3.00 to 8.72, ($p < 0.00001$) and left ventricular ejection fraction (LVEF) decline RR 1.83; 90% CI 1.36 to 2.47 ($p = 0.0008$) [18].

Neoadjuvant chemotherapy is usually indicated either for large operable BC in order to achieve tumor shrinkage enabling these women to have breast conserving surgery, or for locally advanced BC patients to achieve resectability allowing radical mastectomy to be done after successful systemic treatment. In both occasions the systemic therapy is administered with curative intent. Doxo–contained chemotherapy is a part of the majority investigated combinations both in HER2 – negative [19-21] and HER2 - positive BC patients [22, 23]. The definition of pathological complete response (pCR) to neoadjuvant chemotherapy varied across reported studies, but it was achieved in 10 to 20% of HER2-negative BC patients and up to 70% in HER2-positive BC patients when combined with trastuzumab. The most of these studies confirmed that patients who achieve pCR have significantly longer overall survival compared to those w/o pCR at least in triple-negative (TN) and HER2-postiive BC patients, especially in patients younger than 40 years [24].

To conclude, Doxo-containing chemotherapy represents the milestone of (neo)adjuvant therapy in BC patients diagnosed in stage I-III and is recommended by the recent guidelines for the diagnosis and treatment of BC [25, 26]. However, the efficacy of Doxo-containing regimens given in curable stages of BC may be compromised by uncontrolled side effects. Chemotherapy-induced nausea and vomiting (CINV) is one of the most common toxicities related to Doxo administration, especially in combination with cyclophosphamide, which comprises the majority of Doxo-containing (neo)adjuvant regimens. This might preclude BC patients' adherence to therapy, which is proven to significantly prolong overall survival compared to untreated patients [10-year gain of 5%: 39.6% vs. 34.6%; RR 0.84 (95%CI 0.78-0.91), Log-rank $2p<0.00001$] [2]. Hence, the aggressive prevention and treatment of CINV is equally important as antitumor treatment in these patients. Furthermore, cardiotoxicity is an important Doxo-related late side effect which might provoke heart failure and decrease survival at least in some patients. Thus, it is important for clinicians dealing with EBC treatment not to prescribe adjuvant Doxo-containing therapy in patients who would not benefit from it (low-risk patients/luminal A like BC), especially if they are at high risk of developing cardiac complications.

Doxo-Induced Emesis and Vomiting

Pathophysiology of Chemotherapy-Induced Nausea and Vomiting

The mechanisms underlying CINV are not explained in detail yet, but during the last decades considerable improvements have been achieved in our understanding of CINV pathophysiology that led to development of new generations of anti-emetic drugs.

CINV is classified according to time of onset:

- Acute CINV include episodes occurring within a few minutes or several hours after chemotherapy administration, with a maximal intensity after 5-6 hours, and which resolve within 24 hours [27];
- Delayed CINV is defined as those episodes occurring more than 24 hours after chemotherapy, with peaks of intensity generally 48-72 hours after drug administration [28, 29];
- Anticipatory emesis is defined as those episodes that precede drug administration. Since it is a conditioned response, this type of emesis occurs after a previous negative vomiting experience with chemotherapy [30].

Our current knowledge is mainly restricted to interactions between receptors and neurotransmitters responsible for acute CINV, while factors involved in development of delayed CINV are poorly defined.

Mechanisms Responsible for Development of CINV

The best elucidated process involved in development of acute CINV is a vagal-dependent pathway [31]. Initiation of emetic stimuli begins when chemotherapeutic agents, either by direct mucosal or blood-borne mechanisms, provoke exocytotic release of local mediators from enteroendocrine cells placed in the wall of the upper small intestine (Figure 1). At the site of their release, mediators bind to appropriate receptors on vagal afferent terminals, which project to the dorsal brain stem, primarily to the nucleus tractus solitaruis, and, to a lesser extent, the area postrema. Among various local mediators, 5-hydroxytryptamine (5-HT) which binds to 5-HT3 receptors (5-HT3R) is believed to have the most important role in initiation of afferent vagal input. Receptors for other locally released mediators, such as substance P, cholecystokinin, and prostaglandins, are also present on the vagal afferent terminals, but the significance of their assignment at this peripheral site is unknown.

The second possible source of afferent input is the area postrema, where the contribution in CINV is confirmed but exact mechanisms remain to be investigated in detail. The area postrema, also named “chemoreceptor trigger zone", is a circumventricular structure located at the caudal end of the fourth ventricle. It is situated outside of the blood-brain barrier, which makes it accessible to various emetic substances brought by either blood or cerebrospinal fluid. It was shown in animal models that opioids and dopaminergic agonists can induce emetic response, while 5-HT3R antagonists can inhibit cisplatin-induced emesis when they are injected into the area postrema [32, 33]. Though it is highly possible that gut-derived peptides and metabolites of chemotherapeutic agents also can induce emesis by binding at this site, such potential mechanisms remain to be investigated and confirmed.

Afferent stimuli from both described sources are further projected to the final common pathway named "vomiting center" [34]. The vomiting center is located in the medulla and does not exist as a distinct anatomical formation, but rather is a number of loosely organized neuronal areas that coordinate interactions between afferent stimuli and motor outputs by a variety of brainstem nuclei such as the nucleus tractussolitarius, the parvicellular reticular formation, and the Botzinger complex [35, 36]. In addition to the vagal-dependent pathway and area postrema, there are two additional sources of afferent inputs to the vomiting center. The first of them imply direct stimuli from structures in the limbic forebrain, which may be responsible for anticipatory emesis in some patients [37, 38]. The other arises from the vestibular system, but the role of this pathway is less established in CINV.

Neurotransmitters and Receptors

The variety of neurotransmitters and receptors that have been identified within the area postrema and nuclei of the vomiting center has improved our understanding of physiologic mechanisms underlying CINV and has driven significant progress in its treatment. So far, investigations toward control of the emetic reflex have been focused on several neurotransmitters, which have been approved as clinically relevant in the development of CINV, such as dopamine, 5-HT, and substance P, which bind to dopamine D2 receptors (D2R), 5-HT3R, and neurokinin-1R, respectively.

Among the first agents used as antiemetics are drugs that block dopamine D2R. These receptors are found in the area postrema, and their stimulation has been shown to induce emesis in animal models [35]. Dopamine antagonists such as phenothiazines and butyrophenones have been in use for more than forty years in treatment of CINV [39].

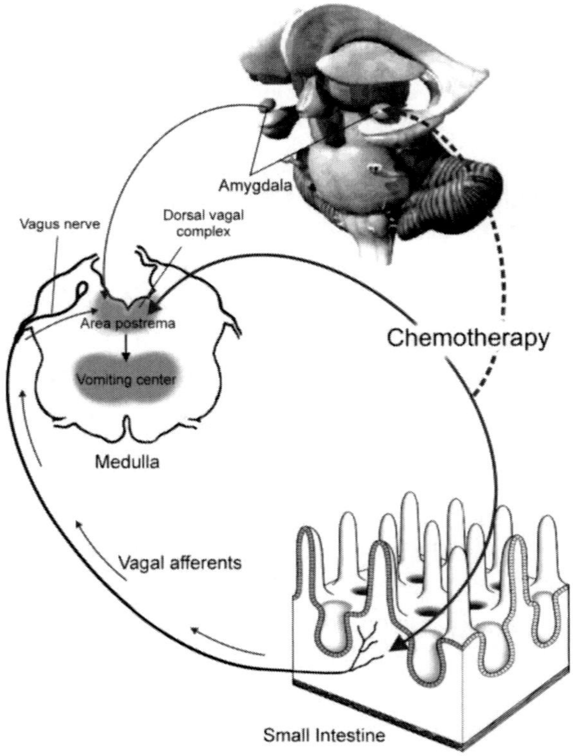

Figure 1. Schematic illustration of chemotherapy-induced emetic response. Chemotherapeutic agents initiate emetic stimuli by two mechanisms. The first mechanism implies direct provocation of exocytotic release of local mediators from enteroendocrine cells placed in the wall of the upper small intestine. Released mediators bind to the receptors on the vagal afferent terminals which project to the dorsal vagal complex and area postrema. The second mechanism includes direct interaction of chemotherapeutic agents, its metabolites or gut-delivered peptides with the area postrema, which is located outside of the blood-brain barrier and accessible to various emetic stimuli brought either by blood or cerebrospinal fluid. Other potential sources of afferent inputs involve a number of structures in the temporal lobe, such as the amygdala, and may be responsible for anticipatory emesis in some patients. Afferent stimuli from all described sources are further projected to the final common pathway named "vomiting center", which coordinates interactions between afferent stimuli and motor outputs by a variety of brainstem nuclei.

Due to their role in initiation of afferent input within the vagal-dependent pathway as well as central localization in area postrema and nucleus tractus solitarius, 5-HT3R and their main agonist 5-HT appear to be most important in regulation of the acute phase of CINV [40, 41]. Although the precise mechanisms of 5-HT involvement in treatment-related emesis are incompletely elucidated, there is strong evidence suggesting antagonism of 5-HT binding to 5-HT3R on vagal afferents rather than in central sites as the dominant mechanism by which 5-HT3R antagonists exert their antiemetic effect [42].

Substance P is the latest recognized, but not least important, neurotransmitter implicated in development of acute and delayed CINV [43]. Together with neurokinin A and neurokinin B substance P makes a group of peptides known as tachykinins, which serve a number of regulatory functions [44]. Substance P binds to receptors neurokinin-1 (NK1R), which has similar distribution to 5-HT3R [45], but contrary to the latter, NK-1R antagonists are effective exclusively on the level of the central nervous system [46].

There are differences in the relative importance of the various neurotransmitters between acute and delayed CINV. Thus, D2R and 5-HT3R antagonists are useful mainly in episodes of acute CINV while they have limited clinical utility in delayed CINV. On the other side, substance P may have the most important role in the pathophysiology of delayed emesis, which is strongly supported by the unique clinical efficacy of the neurokinin-1 antagonists in the delayed emesis settings [47].

Anti-Emetic Prophylaxis for the Combination of Doxo and Cyclophosphamide in Treatment of BC Patients

The risk of developing CINV is fundamentally dependent on the type, dose, schedule and route of administration of chemotherapeutic agents. According to their emetogenic potential, these drugs are divided into 4 groups: highly emetogenic chemotherapy (HEC), which causes emesis in more than 90% of patients, moderately emetogenic chemotherapy (MEC), which causes emesis in 30-90% of patients, and drugs with low and minimal emetogenic potential with 10%-30% and <10% of affected patients, respectively [48, 49].

However, related risk factors of patients, such as sex and age (younger women being particularly at higher risk of developing CINV), prior history of CINV, emesis during pregnancy or motion sickness, alcohol use, tumor burden, anxiety, concomitant medication and medical conditions and inadequate hydration should not be ignored [49] considering they may enhance the emetogenic potential of some drugs or drug combinations. Doxo and cyclophosphamide belong to a group of moderately emetogenic agents, but the combination of these two drugs given to women with BC has been recognized as a special situation with a particularly great risk of nausea and vomiting [50] requiring more aggressive antiemetic regimens [51-53]. Data from previous placebo-controlled studies showed that vomiting occurred in 85% of patients receiving this combination without antiemetic prophylaxis [54].

Antagonists inhibiting the action of neurotransmitters involved in the emetogenic pathway through a blockade of their receptors are widely used as prophylaxis for acute and delayed CINV. Setrons, 5-HT3R antagonists, were introduced in clinical practice more than 20 years ago. Today there are 5 such drugs available: ondansetron, granisetron, dolasetron, tropisetron and palonosetron. Recently published meta-analysis confirmed that palonosetron given before administration of HEC/MEC had a superior effect in alleviating both acute and delayed nausea and vomiting compared to ondansetron, granisetron and dolasetron [55]. Patients receiving palonosetron had less nausea, both acute ($RR = 0.86$; CI $95\% = 0.76$ to 0.96; $p = 0.007$) and delayed ($RR = 0.82$; CI$95\% = 0.75$ to 0.89; $p < 0.00001$) and less acute vomiting ($RR = 0.76$; CI $95\% = 0.66$ to 0.88; $p = 0.0002$) and delayed vomiting ($RR = 0.76$; CI$95\% = 0.68$ to 0.85; $p < 0.00001$). Palonosetron was superior regardless of concomitant corticosteroid use.

Antagonist of NK1R, aprepitant, at first appeared to improve antiemetic prophylaxis for HEC in addition to 5-HT3R antagonists and corticosteroids, has also been shown to do so in BC patients treated with the combination of Doxo and cyclophosphamide [56]. The primary objective of this study was to compare complete remission (CR) rates in two arms. CR was defined as no vomiting and no rescue antiemetics used in the treatment period of 120 days after the administration of chemotherapy. The study confirmed the superiority of the combination of aprepitant, ondansetron and dexamethason in achieving CR in comparison with ondansetron and dexamethason (51% vs. 42%). However, the use of a rescue antiemetic either within the first 24 hours, or after that was the same in both patients groups (59% vs. 56%, NS), implicating that the nausea is not better controlled with aprepitant. Of note, more women in the aprepitant group reported minimal or no impact of emesis on daily life (63.5% v 55.6%; $p=0.019$) measured by the Functional Living Index – Emesis (FLIE) questionnaire. Three-drug regiment was also well tolerated.

In another small non-randomized study, the three-drug regimen consisted of aprepitant, palonosetron and dexamethason given once before the administration of Doxo and cyclophosphamide chemotherapy in BC patients, showed promising results: 51% of patients achieved CR (no vomiting and no rescue antiemetic), 76% in the acute period and 66% in the delayed study period (24-120 hours after chemotherapy). These results confirmed that satisfied emesis protection could be achieved with more convenient single-day antiemetic support [57].

Recently reported results on a randomized study comparing efficacy and tolerability of NEPA (a single oral fixed-dose of netupitant, a new NK1R antagonist and palonosetron, 5-HT3R inhibitor) and dexamethason with standard three-drug regimen consisted of aprepitant, palonosetron and dexamethason in patients receiving HEC and MEC, including the combination of Doxo and cyclophosphamide [58]. The antiemetic regimens were tested in multiple cycles of chemotherapy. Considering that about 40% of included patients completed 6 cycles of chemotherapy this study provide the most information of any multiple cycle antiemetic study. The results revealed that the side effect profiles of both antiemetic regimens were low and comparable. Furthermore, NEPA was shown to be highly effective in preventing CINV following multiple cycles of HEC/MEC (CR were achieved in 81% to 91% of patients throughout the whole study period), and because convenient drug administration offers the opportunity to improve adherence to the CINV prophylaxis guideline.

In short, recently released guidelines for prophylaxis of acute and delayed CINV recognized higher emetogenic potential of the combination of Doxo and cyclophosphamide than each of these drugs exerts [48, 50, 52, 53] in women treated for BC. In line with this statement, three-drug regimen consisting of aprepitant (or fosaprepitant), 5-HT3 antagonist and dexamethason administered on day 1, before chemotherapy is given, is recommended for the prevention of acute CINV, while aprepitant for day 2 and 3 (or nothing if fosaprepitant is given on day 1) is indicated for the prevention of delayed CINV [50]. If NK1R antagonist is not available, than palonosetron is the preferred 5HT3R antagonist.

Unfortunately, CINV is often underestimated by physicians, especially the delayed nausea and vomiting. Being a distinct side effect, it is important to continuously assess nausea and vomiting using reliable tools (visual analogue scale or numerical scale) for measuring the intensity of symptoms [59]. It is also very important for the medical oncologist to adhere to current antiemetic guidelines because acute and delayed CINV may significantly deteriorate patients' quality of lives and influence the patients' non-adherence to otherwise efficacious chemotherapy. Uncontrolled emesis raised the risk of developing the anticipatory emesis which is a major challenge for successful CINV treatment. The best prophylaxis for anticipatory emesis is well controlled CINV from the very beginning of chemotherapy treatment [50].

DOXO-INDUCED CARDIOTOXICITY

Mechanisms of Doxo-Induced Cardiotoxicity

Doxo is a nonselective class I anthracycline, possessing aglyconic and sugar moieties. The aglycone is comprised of a tetracyclic ring with quinine-hydroquinone adjacent groups, methoxy substituent short side chain followed by the carbonyl group. The sugar component (also known as daunosamine) is attached to one of the rings by a glycosidic bond.

Although Doxo cardiotoxic activity has been recognized over 4 decades ago, mechanisms underlying cardiotoxicity are still a matter of controversy. Several hypotheses are offered to explain Doxo-induced cardiotoxicity, but neither of them adequately integrates clinical manifestations with existing basic science knowledge.

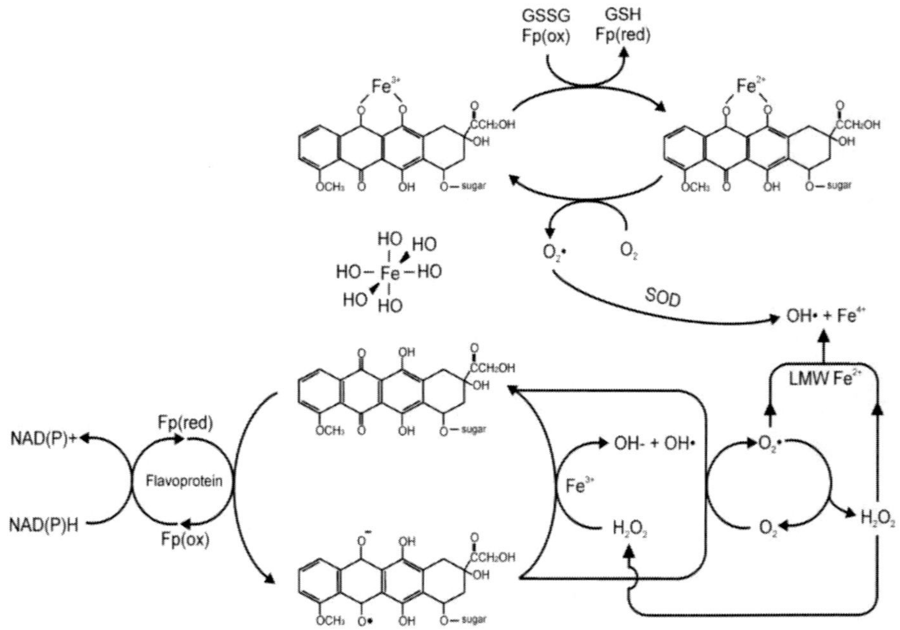

Figure 2. Schematic illustration of doxorubicin-induced oxidative stress production. Non-enzymatic (above) and enzymatic (below) mechanisms by which doxorubicin generates free radicals. Fp, flavoprotein; NAD(P)H, nicotinamide adenine dinucleotide (phosphate); LMW, low molecular weight; GSH, glutathione; GSSG, glutathione disulfide; SOD, superoxide dismutase.

Free radical hypothesis

Biochemical and physiological data favor the hypothesis that the general antineoplastic cytotoxicity of anthracyclines relies on the formation of reactive oxygen species (ROS) whose intermediates interact with and damage cellular membranes [60]. Two mechanisms responsible for generation of ROS are described: non-enzymatic and enzymatic (Figure 2).

The non-enzymatic mechanism involves interaction of iron(III) with ketone and hydroxyl groups positioned on C-11 and C-12 atoms of Doxo, which induces an internal redox reaction wherein an electron flows from the C-14 hydroxyl group to iron, generating an iron (II)-Doxo free radical complex [61]. This complex further reduces oxygen to superoxide anion (O•), after which an electron flows from iron(II) to Doxo, resulting in an iron(III)-Doxo free radical complex. Afterwards, the iron(III)-Doxo free radical complex rearranges to iron(II)-Doxo (aldehyde), which becomes oxidized to iron(III)-Doxo (aldehyde) as another molecule of oxygen is reduced to O•.

Enzymatic mechanism involves anthracycline quinine moiety, which can be reduced to a semiquinone due to single electron reduction from donors such as NADPH and NADH in reaction, which is catalized by cytochrome P-450 reductase. Once formed, semiquinone, as it cycles back to the quinine, transfers an electron to molecular oxygen, generating superoxide anion (O•) and its dismutation product hydrogen peroxide (H_2O_2), increasing these species above physiological levels generated during normal aerobic metabolism [62].

Oxidative stress induced by generated ROS alters the structure and function of lipid components that act as precursors of second messengers [63]. ROS readily reacts with a variety of molecules and causes peroxidation of membrane lipids, resulting in membrane degradation, protein aggregation, and cell death [64, 65]. Body of evidence indicates that the major products of lipid peroxidation are a great variety of stable, diffusible saturated and unsaturated aldehydes. The cytotoxic aldehydes are extremely active, they can diffuse within or even escape from the cell and attack targets far from the site of the original free radical initiated event, and therefore act as “second cytotoxic messengers” [66-68]. Aldehydes are potent cytotoxic agents that react with different biomolecules, thus changing the biochemical status of the cell, finally resulting in cell damage [69]. The concentration of aldehydes in rat plasma and heart tissue increased significantly following in vivo Doxo treatment. The changes occurred early, peaked around 2 hours after Doxo administration, and the levels declined or returned to normal values within 8-24 hours [70].

Because heart cells are so rich in heme-containing proteins that may undergo auto-oxidation, the presence of excess intracellular peroxide in the anthracycline-treated heart would establish an extraordinarily favorable milieu for the formation of highly reactive hydroxyl and peroxy radicals with a proven capacity to produce membrane peroxidation [71]. Both O• and H_2O_2 have their inherent toxicity, but cell damage ensues more rapidly when they react with low molecular weight (LMW) iron [72], which in physiological conditions is stored within an iron-containing protein complex called ferritin. However, there are two mechanisms by which Doxo can release iron from ferritin. The first of them involves O•, which is small enough to penetrate the transprotein channels of ferritin and has a reduction potential lower than that of ferritin-bounded iron. The other one implies the semiquinone ring of Doxo, which can release iron by virtue of the electrontunneling mechanism, which are relayed by redox sites on the surface and transprotein channels of ferritin. Such released LMW Fe(II) can decompose H_2O_2 into highly reactive hydroxyl radicals (•OH), or can be converted by H_2O_2 into ferryl ions having the same reactivity as •OH [73]. Both ferryl ions and •OH can eventually cause cardiac dysfunction by oxidizing lipids, proteins, and DNA.

There was significant experimental data that raised suspicions about the strength of free radical hypothesis [60], which initiated other attempts to explain the mechanism of Doxo cardiotoxicity. Also, with an attempt to explain the lack of protection by antioxidants, one might argue that free radical processes are more a consequence than a cause of tissue damage. In apparent support of this hypothesis, antioxidants such as α-tocopherol and N-acetylcisteine have been shown to reduce Doxo-induced cardiomyopathy in Doxo-treated tumor-free animals [74, 75], but in clinical trials progressive decline of cardiac functions was not prevented by supplementing patients with either of these two antioxidants [76]. Also, it was indicated that cardiac lipid peroxidation proceeds via reactive intermediates and must be different from the hydroxyl radical since it cannot promote lipid peroxidation since it exhibits a diffusion-limited reactivity and cannot migrate from the site of generation to the hydrophobic membrane phases where the bis-allylic bonds are buried [73].

There are a few offered explanations which have been brought to focus when the group of authors unraveled "free radical paradox" in the sense that cancer patients have a spontaneous exacerbation of cardiac lipid peroxidation, which is actually abolished by Doxo treatments [77]. One possibility is that anthracyclines form too many radicals, setting the stage for radical-radical interactions that eventually extinguish oxidative stress. Thus, semiquinone free radicals might terminate lipid peroxidation by preferentially interacting with lipid radical species rather than with oxygen or iron [78]. On the other side, it was suggested that oxidative damage could be abolished due to unbalanced Fe(II):Fe(III) ratio when free radicals generate H_2O_2 in excess of Fe(II), causing the oxidation of Fe(II) and shifting the Fe(II)/Fe(III) ration toward the unreactive Fe(III) [73]. Similar consideration has been extended with the catalase study, where higher levels of catalase expression did not prevent, but enhanced lipid peroxidation [79]. These studies indirectly confirm that free radical injury is promoted when Fe(II) is "protected" from excessive oxidation by H_2O_2, which presumably occurs at very high levels of enzyme expression.

Since ROS are very short-lived species, their presence is closely linked to the presence of their generating source in the tissue, which makes it unlikely that they are directly responsible for the delayed cardiotoxic phase. Therefore, the development of Doxo-induced cardiotoxicity must be due to a complex sequence of events in which the presence of Doxo is required only at the beginning to initiate the process.

Calcium overload hypothesis and role of mitochondrion

According to this theory, Doxo causes excessive levels of intracellular calcium, which leads to mitochondrial dysfunction, depletion of high-energy phosphates, increased muscle stiffness, contractile dysfunction, and cell death. However, works of Jensen [80] and Rabkin [81] provided evidences that calcium accumulation may be a manifestation rather than a cause of Doxo cardiomyopathy suggesting that Doxo-induced cardiac dysfunction is associated with a deficiency rather than an excess of calcium at the myofibrillar apparatus. Doxo-induced inhibition of mitochondrial calcium accumulation had been widely documented [82, 83], while Solem and Wallace [84] provided evidence for specific action of Doxo on the ADP/ATP antiport, independent of the uptake uniport and the isoelectric sodium-calcium antiport.

The direct effect of Doxo on mitochondrial structure and function has been confirmed by various morphological and biochemical effects, including histopathological changes as swelling and vacuolization of the mitochondria as early characteristics of Doxo therapy [85], impaired respiration [86], inhibition of coenzyme Q-dependent enzymes [87], decreased oxidative activity [88], swelling and lysis [89], increased inner membrane permeability [86], depletion of glutathione and enhanced lipid peroxidation [90], and formation of strong electrostatic complexes with cardiolipin associated with the inner membrane [91]. The inner mitochondrial membrane, which houses the enzymes of the electron transfer chain (ETC), possesses a particularly high content of cardiolipins, which are essential to the subunit assembly and catalytic function of these proteins [92, 93]. Doxo has been shown to have a high affinity for cardiolipin and inhibition of the complexes of II-IV activity, and this impact on the ETC results from an alteration in the membrane organization rather than direct protein interaction [94, 95]. However, association with the mitochondrial membrane environment likely situates Doxo in close proximity to complex I, which serves as the reductive enzyme, which results in the mitochondrion electron transport producing the majority of the ROS from Doxo redox cycling in the heart [96-98]. Evidence for elevated ROS generation subsequent to Doxo treatment is included in studies on rats, where ROS generation was continually increasing for 5 weeks compared to 1 week after treatment was terminated [99].

Doxo metabolite hypothesis

Studies with myocardial fragments disposed during aorto-coronary bypass grafting demonstrated that cytosolic fraction from human myocardium posses NADPH-dependent aldo-ketoreductases that add two electrons to the C-13 carbonyl group in the side chain of Doxo, forming a second alcohol metabolite called doxorubicinol (DoxOL) [100]. From a pharmacokinetic viewpoint, DoxOL would seem more likely than Doxo to mediate the delayed cardiotoxicity of Doxo treatment. DoxOL, but not Doxo, has been observed to accumulate in cardiac tissue. For example, DoxOL concentrations in rat heart reached the highest values after the last of three weekly injections of Doxo in doses of 2 mg/kg [101].

DoxOL is a potent inhibitor of the specific ion-dependent pumps of sarcoplasmic reticulum (SR), mitochondria, and sarcolemma [102, 103]. Those effects are probably unrelated to free radical production because DoxOL inhibits these enzyme activities more rapidly than can be accounted for free radical mechanism. DoxOL can therefore affect myocardial energy metabolism, ionic gradients, and Ca^{2+} movements, ultimately impairing cardiac contraction and relaxation. Further investigations showed that DoxOL irreversibly inactivates cytosolic aconitase/IRP1, which is a bifunctional protein that modulates iron uptake versus sequestration thus regulating the concentration of metabolically available LMW Fe [104].

Hypothesis on inhibition of DNA, RNA and protein synthesis

Different hypotheses have been proposed to explain delayed cardiotoxicity, and most of them were based on an initial selective DNA lesion by Doxo, which would lead to inhibition of the synthesis of critical proteins or enzymes. This theory is supported by the observation that one-electron reduction of Doxo can occur in the nuclear envelope [105] as well as the mitochondria, and that DNA breakdown is produced by Doxo in the presence of transition metals, particularly iron [106]. If the turnover rate of target biomolecules were slow, overt cardiotoxicity would only develop when resynthesis of the involved biomolecules is required.

Kurabayashi and colleagues [107-109] have demonstrated that within several hours Doxo dramatically and selectively suppresses the expression of several nuclear genes, which encode enzymes that play central roles in normal energy production. One of these genes encodes the heart- and muscle-specific isoform of ADP/ATP translocase (ANT1), the second encodes the Reiske iron-sulfur (RISK) protein, which is a ubiquitously expressed component of the ETC, and third encodes M isoenzyme of the critical metabolic enzyme 6-phosphofructo-1-kinase (PFK). The rapid changes in ATP production that would follow from reduction of these key metabolic enzymatic activities might well be more central to the effect of the antharcycline drugs.

Another study showed that the mRNA expression levels for proteins that controlled the release and uptake of Ca^{2+} through the sarcoplasmic reticulum (SR) membrane such as ryanodine receptor (required for Ca^{2+} release), SERCA2 and phospholamban (regulate Ca^{2+} uptake) and calsequestrin (manages Ca^{2+} storage) were reduced in the failing hearts of the animals subjected to Doxo administration [110]. On the other side, levels of mRNA for membrane Ca^{2+} transport were unaffected by Doxo treatment, which was in correlation with the ultramicroscopic observation that transverse tubules appear normal despite the involvement of SR in the damaged myocytes [111]. Ito et al. [112] demonstrated that Doxo selectively decreased the levels of mRNA for the sarcomeric genes, α-actin, troponin I, myosin light chain 2, and the muscle-specific isoforms of creatine kinase, pyruvate kinase or β-actin, indicating that Doxo has an apparent selectivity to inhibit transcription of genes expressed in muscle cells.

Prevention and Management of Doxo-Induced Cardiotoxicity

After intravenous infusion, Doxo undergoes a triphasic plasma clearance. It is distributed in the tissues rapidly with a half-life of 3-5 minutes, while its terminal half-life of 24-36 hours suggests that Doxo takes far longer to be eliminated from the tissue than its uptake [113]. The range of steady distribution is from 500-800 L/m^2, which allows all tissues to take up a potent amount of Doxo. Doxo binds to plasma proteins and enters the cell via passive diffusion, with intracellular accumulation that exceed the extracellular compartment by 10- to 500-fold. Within the cell, the mitochondria and nucleus have been shown to effectively accumulate the drug [114, 115]. In the organism Doxo undergoes modification by several enzymes, predominantly in the liver [116], and its metabolites include an alcohol produced via carbonyl reduction (DoxOL) and several aglycone derivatives. It is excreted mostly through the feces in the DoxOL and parent form, suggesting that conversion to metabolites is not extensive [117]. In the human heart, both alcohol and the parent form are the most prominent [118]. Doxo cannot pass the brain-blood barrier.

Assessment of subclinical damage of myocardial tissue is based on the imaging techniques like echocardiography, MST, NMR and MUGA. All of these imaging techniques assess the ejection fraction of the left ventricle (LVEF), which is the most important determinant of the heart function. In different studies the measurement of decline in LVEF was defined in different ways, but in recent work of Curigliano et al., this issue is resolved by the definition that the decline in LVEF of at least 5% to less than 55% with the accompanying signs or symptoms of chronic heart failure, or a decline in LVEF of at least 10% to below 55% without accompanying signs or symptoms, was referred to as a significant damage [119].

Acute effects of Doxo cardiotoxic activity are characterized by a variety of acute atrial and ventricular dysrhythmias, a pericarditis-myocarditis syndrome, and acute hypertensive reactions occurring shortly after administration of the drug, which are usually transient and clinically manageable [120]. Acute heart failure and even myocardial infarction may be one of the cardiotoxic manifestations. On rare occasions, sudden cardiac death also occurred [121]. The long-term effects include concealed onset of cardiomyopathy, which often leads to congestive heart failure. These late manifestations of Doxo cardiotoxicity often develop after months, sometimes even years after therapy has been completed. Morphologic abnormalities of Doxo-induced cardiomyopathy include the loss of myofibrils, dilation of the sarcoplasmic reticulum, cytoplasmic vacuolization, swelling of mitochondria, increased number of lysosomes, atrophy of myocytes, and interstitial edema and fibrosis [122-124].

Correlation between the dose of Doxo and the risk of cardiomyopathy and congestive heart failure (CHF) has been established in a seminal retrospective study on 399 patient records [89]. In another retrospective review of several thousand patients receiving Doxo-containing chemotherapy, the risk of CHF correlated with patient age, total dose, and dose schedule [125]. Younger patients are subject to higher risk, with 25% of them <15 years old showing CHF after 450 mg/m^2 Doxo and the incidence increasing linearly above 550 mg/m^2. Approximately half of all patients receiving ≥1000 mg/m^2 experience CHF [125]. Long-term follow-up studies suggest that cardiotoxicity occurs in as many as 71% of patients treated with anthracyclines as children [126]. Valvular, coronary, or myocardial heart disease and a long-standing history of hypertension were recognized as independent risk factors of developing cardiomyopathy at cumulative doses of Doxo below 500 to 550 mg/m^2. Previous mediastinal irradiation or concurrent administration of other chemotherapeutics (e.g., cyclophosphamide) was also considered to increase the risk [125]. If a lifetime accumulation of Doxo nears 500 mg/m^2, the risk of cardiomyopathy increases often resulting in CHF in 20% of patients. While the probability of cardiotoxicity is clearly related to cumulative dose, it is important to remember that the cardiac effects of these drugs start from the first dose. Thus, CHF has been reported after a single 50 mg/m^2 dose of Doxo [125].

Strategies for Prevention of Doxo-Induced Cardiotoxicity

Slow infusion

Continuous infusion of Doxo over 48 to 96 hours rather than the standard 15 minutes bolus proved to be an effective method to reduce severe morphologic changes in endomyocardial biopsies and the development of clinically evident CHF, while not diminishing tumor objective response in patients receiving cumulative doses of 600 mg/m^2 [127]. Because cardiotoxic activity of Doxo appears to correlate with the first peak plasma level, but not the area under the curve, the safety and efficacy of replacing the bolus administration with slow infusion have been confirmed [128]. In agreement with this, studies with rabbits showed that both plasma and left ventricular peak plasma concentrations of Doxo and DoxOL were significantly higher following bolus slow infusion [129]. However, this method is not widely accepted because it requires a central venous catheter or a pump, which is inconvenient for the patient, and carries the risk of infection.

Drug delivery systems

Development of new drug delivery systems has been initiated by a quest for a solution, which would provide targeted tumor delivery with reduced non-tumor toxicity due to a modified pharmacokinetic profile of the cytotoxic drug.

After initial failure, which implies easy recognition and removal of liposomes from the circulatory system via the reticuloendothelial system (RES) because of composition and size of particles [130], liposomes were soon coated with polyethylene glycol (PEG) to prolong circulation time. PEG liposomes become known as "stealth", one of which eventually commercialized with Doxo. The pharmacokinetic profile of PEG-Doxo liposomes is quite different to Doxo alone. One of the main differences is the smaller volume of distribution and clearance rate, but most importantly, those particles hold the potential to be delivered selectively at tumor sites owing to their small size (about 100 nm), which allows them to penetrate through defective blood vessels supplying the tumor [131]. Studies conducted in rats with brain implanted sarcoma showed that the PEG-Doxo liposomes thoroughly penetrated the intracerebral tumors at the same time sparing the surrounding healthy brain tissue, depicting a critical advantage over free Doxo [132].

Another step forward was the introduction of nanoparticles synthesized via an imine reaction between oxidized dextran and polyethylene-imine (PEI) of a low molecular weight [133]. One such example produced dextran-graft-PEI nanoparticles loaded with Doxo [134]. Nevertheless, these products have not yet found a place in routine practice since there is a need for more long-term data regarding their efficacy and toxicity, as well as the high cost of these products.

Antioxidants

The great part of strategies focused on protection from Doxo cardiotoxicity were relying on administration of drugs, which should improve the antioxidant defense of the heart against anthracycline-derived ROS. Most frequently investigated antioxidants include probucol (a lipid-lowering drug), piperidinenitroxides, lipophilic spin traps, melatonin, vitamins A, E and C, and thiol-containing agents [135-139]. The advantage of these compounds was that these agents did not interfere with activity of anthracyclines in tumor cells, which supported hopes for pharmacologic interventions that improved the therapeutic index of anthracyclines. Unfortunately, cardioprotective efficacy of antioxidants like vitamin E and N-acetylcysteine was disappointing in large-sized animals such as dogs and pigs, while in clinical studies these two agents neither prevented nor delayed the development of cardiomyopathy in patients treated with cumulative doses of anthracyclines [138, 140].

Among antioxidant agents, amifostine has attracted more attention since it is a thiophosphate, which in its active form contains free thiol that may act as a scavenger of free radicals generated in tissue exposed to cytotoxic drugs, and binds to active metabolites of such drugs. It was originally developed as a radioprotective agent in a classified nuclear warfare project, and after the project had been declassified, amifostine was introduced in evaluation as a cytoprotective agent against toxicity of alkylating drugs and cisplatin. As a pro-drug, amifostine is dephosphorylated by a membrane-bound alkaline phosphatase, which is a transformation that occurs in normal tissue more effectively than in malignant foci because of impaired alkaline phosphatase activity in tumors due to low pH values found within hypoxic tumor masses [141, 142].

In cultures of rat cardiomyocytes, amifostine significantly increased glutathione levels and reduced Doxo-induced heart-cell toxicity measured by adenosine triphosphate content [143], while on a Langendorff-type model of rat heart amifostine induced a coronary dilatation and displayed a cardioprotective effect when it was administered with cardiotoxic concentrations of Doxo [144]. In vivo investigations on rodents provided contradictory results. In part of these experiments amifostine attenuated Doxo-induced cardiotoxicity [145], decreased Doxo-induced lipid peroxidation with increased levels of the protective enzymes in the heart tissue [146], and significantly improved left ventricular pressure compared to Doxo single-treated animals [147]. On the other side, amifostine did not prevent but only delayed the onset of cardiac lesions [148], while it completely failed in investigation with young rats when amifostine actually increased toxicity and mortality induced by Doxo [149]. In two clinical studies administration of amifostine caused mild to moderate transit side effects including a drop in systolic blood pressure and episodes of nausea/vomiting, but overall conclusion was that amifostine ameliorated Doxo-related toxicity with an improvement in patients' quality of life [150, 151]. Today, amifostine is indicated in patients receiving repeated cisplatin doses for advanced cancer to prevent or reduce renal damage, and to reduce incidence of moderate to severe xerostomia in patients undergoing radiation of the parotid gland for head and neck cancer.

Iron chelators (dexrazoxane)

Dexrazoxane is a bisketopiperazine, originally developed by Creighton et al. as a potential anticancer agent [152], which undergoes stepwise hydrolysis of the two piperazine rings to form one-ring open intermediates. The latter form eventually hydrolyzes to give a diacid-diamide that is structurally reminiscent of EDTA and chelates iron bound to low-molecular-weight cellular ligands or coordinated within 3:1 anthracycline/Fe complexes [153].

Despite intensive research, there is limited data available on mechanisms involved in dexrazoxane-afforded cardioprotection.

In preclinical settings, dexrazoxane prevented damage of cardiomyocytes induced with a wide range of Doxo concentrations, while its metabolites did not lead authors to the conclusion that some other mechanism than iron chelations might be involved in the cardioprotective effect of dexrazoxane [154, 155]. Others have suggested that dexrazoxane may act as a scavenger of ROS without enzymatic hydrolysis and its antioxidant effect may be iron independent [156]. In a study on isolated heart perfused with Doxo, dexrazoxane significantly reduced production of •OH, but this production did not show a common concentration-response relationship with a concentration of dexrazoxane [157]. Furthermore, treatment with dexrazoxane rescued cardiomyocytes from complex pro-apoptotic signaling, but no correlation has been found between myocardial malondialdehyde levels and parameters of cardiac function, as well as protection with dexrazoane was not associated with significantly decreased markers of lipoperoxidation [158]. Moreover, dexrazoxane significantly delayed the development of multidrug resistance, a frequent complication of Doxo chemotherapy [159]. Our results showed that dexrazoxane significantly reduced myocardial injury induced by bolus dose of Doxo, and even more important, it reversed progression of initial pathological changes in time toward dilative cardiomyopathy [160]. Unfortunately, when dexrazoxane was challenged against a combination of Doxo and cyclophosphamide the same level of cardioprotection was not achieved compared to that of a single Doxo treatment [161].

Several clinical trials have demonstrated the cardioprotective effect of dexrazoxane in patients treated with Doxo. As advanced breast cancer accounts for the largest population of patients treated with Doxo, the bulk of the evidence demonstrating cardioprotection with dexrazoxane has been obtained in this group [162-167], where dexrazoxane was co-administered from the first dose in most of these studies. However, early retrospective analysis suggested that dexrazoxane is still effective as a cardioprotectant if administered following a previous cumulative dose of >300 mg/m^2 doxorubicin [168].

Although early preclinical examinations have shown no effect of dexrazoxane on the anticancer activity of Doxo [169], suspicion on this issue has arisen from one of the phase III trials [164]. This has been reflected in recommendations for dexrazoxane use given by various oncological societies, what initiated a meta-analysis of all available data from the randomized trials which demonstrated that control/placebo patients have equivalent tumor responses to patients receiving dexrazoxane [170]. However, in the official FDA information for dexrazoxane it is underlined that, due to results in the largest of three breast cancer trials which showed patients who received dexrazoxane starting with the first cycle of FAC therapy had a lower response rate and shorter time to progression than patients who did not receive it, dexrazoxane should only be used in those patients who have received a cumulative Doxo dose of 300 mg/m^2 and are continuing with Doxo therapy [171]. Another restriction for use of dexrazoxane are results of two open studies which reported a three-fold increase in the incidence of second primary malignancies (particularly acute myeloid leukemia, AML and myelodysplastic syndrome) in dexrazoxane-treated children compared with controls [172, 173]. A significant increase of other toxicities compared with controls, including severe myelosuppression and severe infection, was also reported in one study [174]. According to these results, use of dexrazoxane has been restricted to adults with advanced or metastatic breast cancer who have previously received a minimum cumulative dose of 300 mg/m^2 Doxo. Dexrazoxane is no longer indicated for use in patients with malignancies other than breast cancer, and is contraindicated for use in children and adolescents up to age 18 years because of evidence of serious harm in this age-group [175].

Management of Doxo-Induced Cardiotoxicity

Management of acute Doxo-induced cardiotoxic manifestations

Biochemical monitoring tests that can be used in assessment of acute Doxocardiotoxicity are troponin and brain natriuretic peptide (BNP). These biomarkers are well established indicators of myocardial necrosis and heart failure in different heart diseases, and in recent years they have been extensively studied in settings of cardiotoxicity [176-179]. Most of these studies have shown that the elevation of biomarkers have prognostic value in the development of a late onset of the heart failure. Because we do not have particular studies dealing with arrhythmia in acute cardiotoxicity, treatment of rhythm disturbances in these settings should follow recent guidelines for the treatment of particular arrhythmia. Supraventricular and ventricular rhythm disturbances should be treated with beta blockers like metoprolol, bisoprolol or on some occasions sotalol. Although sotalol is effective in suppressing ventricular rhythm disturbances it has very serious side effects, like pro-arrhythmic properties, and should not be used as the first choice treatment, particularly in chronic therapy. If serious arrhythmia occurred amiodaron can be used [180, 181], and in some cases, one of the treatment modalities is also implantation of implantable cardioverter defibrillators (ICD) [182]. In the case when supraventricular or ventricular arrhythmia induces a chemodynamic compromise, electrical cardio version should be employed. Heart failure in patients with acute cardiotoxicity should be treated according to the guidelines for acute heart failure. They include nitrate and diuretics, and later in the course, beta blockers and angiotensin converting enzyme (ACE) inhibitors [183].

Monitoring and management of late Doxo-induced cardiotoxic manifestations

According to the latest ESMO clinical guidelines [119], patients on doxorubicin treatment should be assessed for troponin (either TrI or TrT) and BNP serum levels after each cycle of doxorubicin therapy and if it becomes positive, therapy with an ACE inhibitor should be started. An echocardiography exam should be performed at three, six and nine months after troponins were determined as positive for the first time.

When the LVEF drops more than 15% from the baseline, but still is in the range of normal values, treatment with Doxo can be continued. But if the LVEF declines below 50% during doxorubicin containing regimens, echocardiography reassessment is mandatory 3 weeks later. If the result of the LVEF is confirmed after 3 weeks, chemotherapy must be held, starting with the therapy for left ventricular dysfunction (LVD), and further frequent clinical and echocardiographic checks.

In the case that LVEF declines less than 40%, current chemotherapy should be discontinued, alternative protocols should be discussed for LVD treatment with enalapril and beta-blockers (preferably carvedilol) if there are no existing contraindications. Patients who start with this therapy early after detection of heart dysfunction have higher chances for recovery of the heart dysfunction within one year. If the treatment for LVD was not initiated within six months after dysfunction is detected, chances for recovery of the heart function are very small [184].

Patients who do not respond to therapy for LVD but progressively continue with declining LVEF should be treated with diuretics, ACE inhibitors or angiotensin receptor blockers (ARB), and beta-blockers in their maximal tolerated doses [183]. Digoxin should be given as a fourth line agent to reduce hospitalization, rhythm disturbances and better exercise tolerance.

When the standard therapy for the heart failure does not improve clinical status of the patient, new device treatments should be considered. In some case reports, the cardiac resynchronization therapy (CRT) device has consistently improved LVEF accompanied by progress in patient subjective response [185, 186], which makes it a valuable option for some patients. However, there are no prospective studies that have investigated the long-term benefit of this treatment modality, but use of CRT device should be evaluated in the setting of Doxo and other chemotherapeutic protocols, which carry increased risk for the development of cardiac dysfunction.

Conclusion

Although Doxo has been used for treating cancer for over 40 years, it still remains one of the most effective anticancer agents. However, its efficacy does not come without a price which includes life-threatening toxicities to most major organs. In case of patients suffering malignancies with short life expectancy, late toxicities of Doxo treatment such as development of CHF or secondary malignancies are less worrisome. On the other side, Doxo-containing chemotherapy represents the milestone of therapy in BC patients diagnosed in stage I-III offering long OS and DFS, which may be discredited by uncontrolled Doxo side effects. Proper handling of CINV during the therapy reduces patient's renouncement due to increased physical and psychological discomfort, while reduced risk of cardiotoxicity provides an uncompromised quality of life and survival benefit. Certain enhancements that we presented here are already used in reducing or managing toxicities. Nevertheless, despite the number of targeted anticancer agents that are already introduced in clinics, the future of the continued use of Doxo in treatment of BC appears to be settled which urges further investigations and innovations toward additional increased safety of Doxo-containing treatments.

References

[1] Polychemotherapy for early breast cancer: an overview of the randomised trials. Early Breast Cancer Trialists' Collaborative Group. *Lancet*, 1998, 352(9132), 930-942.

[2] Effects of chemotherapy and hormonal therapy for early breast cancer on recurrence and 15-year survival: an overview of the randomised trials. *Lancet*, 2005, 365(9472), 1687-1717.

[3] Chia, S; Bryce, C; Gelmon, K. The 2000 EBCTCG overview: a widening gap. *Lancet*, 2005, 365(9472), 1665-1666.

[4] Peto, R; Davies, C; Godwin, J; Gray, R; Pan, HC; Clarke, M; et al. Comparisons between different polychemotherapy regimens for early breast cancer: meta-analyses of long-term outcome among 100,000 women in 123 randomised trials. *Lancet*, 2012, 379(9814), 432-444.

[5] Pritchard, KI; Shepherd, LE; O'Malley, FP; Andrulis, IL; Tu, D; Bramwell, VH; et al. HER2 and responsiveness of breast cancer to adjuvant chemotherapy. *N. Engl. J. Med.*, 2006, 354(20), 2103-2111.

[6] Hutchins, LF; Green, SJ; Ravdin, PM; Lew, D; Martino, S; Abeloff, M; et al. Randomized, controlled trial of cyclophosphamide, methotrexate, and fluorouracil versus cyclophosphamide, doxorubicin, and fluorouracil with and without tamoxifen for high-risk, node-negative breast cancer: treatment results of Intergroup Protocol INT-0102. *J. Clin. Oncol.*, 2005, 23(33), 8313-8321.

[7] Bernard-Marty, C; Mano, M; Paesmans, M; Accettura, C; Munoz-Bermeo, R; Richard, T; et al. Second malignancies following adjuvant chemotherapy: 6-year results from a Belgian randomized study comparing cyclophosphamide, methotrexate and 5-fluorouracil (CMF) with an anthracycline-based regimen in adjuvant treatment of node-positive breast cancer patients. *Ann. Oncol.*, 2003, 14(5), 693-698.

[8] Conforti, R; Boulet, T; Tomasic, G; Taranchon, E; Arriagada, R; Spielmann, M; et al. Breast cancer molecular subclassification and estrogen receptor expression to predict efficacy of adjuvant anthracyclines-based chemotherapy: a biomarker study from two randomized trials. *Ann. Oncol.*, 2007, 18(9), 1477-1483.

[9] Berry, DA; Cirrincione, C; Henderson, IC; Citron, ML; Budman, DR; Goldstein, LJ; et al. Estrogen-receptor status and outcomes of modern chemotherapy for patients with node-positive breast cancer. *JAMA*, 2006, 295(14), 1658-1667.

[10] Albain, KS; Barlow, WE; Shak, S; Hortobagyi, GN; Livingston, RB; Yeh, IT; et al. Prognostic and predictive value of the 21-gene recurrence score assay in postmenopausal women with node-positive, oestrogen-receptor-positive breast cancer on chemotherapy: a retrospective analysis of a randomised trial. *Lancet Oncol.*, 2010, 11(1), 55-65.

[11] Andre, F; Broglio, K; Roche, H; Martin, M; Mackey, JR; Penault-Llorca, F; et al. Estrogen receptor expression and efficacy of docetaxel-containing adjuvant chemotherapy in patients with node-positive breast

cancer: results from a pooled analysis. *J. Clin. Oncol.*, 2008, 26(16), 2636-2643.

[12] Coates, AS; Colleoni, M; Goldhirsch, A. Is adjuvant chemotherapy useful for women with luminal a breast cancer? *J. Clin. Oncol.*, 2012, 30(12), 1260-1263.

[13] Henderson, IC; Berry, DA; Demetri, GD; Cirrincione, CT; Goldstein, LJ; Martino, S; et al. Improved outcomes from adding sequential Paclitaxel but not from escalating Doxorubicin dose in an adjuvant chemotherapy regimen for patients with node-positive primary breast cancer. *J. Clin. Oncol.*, 2003, 21(6), 976-983.

[14] Citron, ML; Berry, DA; Cirrincione, C; Hudis, C; Winer, EP; Gradishar, WJ; et al. Randomized trial of dose-dense versus conventionally scheduled and sequential versus concurrent combination chemotherapy as postoperative adjuvant treatment of node-positive primary breast cancer: first report of Intergroup Trial C9741/Cancer and Leukemia Group B Trial 9741. *J. Clin. Oncol.*, 2003, 21(8), 1431-1439.

[15] Slamon, D; Eiermann, W; Robert, N; Pienkowski, T; Martin, M; Press, M; et al. Adjuvant trastuzumab in HER2-positive breast cancer. *N. Engl. J. Med.*, 2011, 365(14), 1273-1283.

[16] Perez, EA; Romond, EH; Suman, VJ; Jeong, JH; Davidson, NE; Geyer, CE, Jr.; et al. Four-year follow-up of trastuzumab plus adjuvant chemotherapy for operable human epidermal growth factor receptor 2-positive breast cancer: joint analysis of data from NCCTG N9831 and NSABP B-31. *J. Clin. Oncol.*, 2011, 29(25), 3366-3373.

[17] Gianni, L; Dafni, U; Gelber, RD; Azambuja, E; Muehlbauer, S; Goldhirsch, A; et al. Treatment with trastuzumab for 1 year after adjuvant chemotherapy in patients with HER2-positive early breast cancer: a 4-year follow-up of a randomised controlled trial. *Lancet Oncol.*, 2011, 12(3), 236-244.

[18] Moja, L; Tagliabue, L; Balduzzi, S; Parmelli, E; Pistotti, V; Guarneri, V; et al. Trastuzumab containing regimens for early breast cancer. *Cochrane. Database. Syst. Rev.*, 2012, 4CD006243-

[19] von, MG; Raab, G; Caputo, A; Schutte, M; Hilfrich, J; Blohmer, JU; et al. Doxorubicin with cyclophosphamide followed by docetaxel every 21 days compared with doxorubicin and docetaxel every 14 days as preoperative treatment in operable breast cancer: the GEPARDUO study of the German Breast Group. *J. Clin. Oncol.*, 2005, 23(12), 2676-2685.

[20] Bear, HD; Anderson, S; Smith, RE; Geyer, CE, Jr.; Mamounas, EP; Fisher, B; et al. Sequential preoperative or postoperative docetaxel

added to preoperative doxorubicin plus cyclophosphamide for operable breast cancer:National Surgical Adjuvant Breast and Bowel Project Protocol B-27. *J. Clin. Oncol.*, 2006, 24(13), 2019-2027.

[21] von, MG; Kummel, S; Vogel, P; Hanusch, C; Eidtmann, H; Hilfrich, J; et al. Intensified neoadjuvant chemotherapy in early-responding breast cancer: phase III randomized GeparTrio study. *J. Natl. Cancer Inst.*, 2008, 100(8), 552-562.

[22] Gianni, L; Eiermann, W; Semiglazov, V; Manikhas, A; Lluch, A; Tjulandin, S; et al. Neoadjuvant chemotherapy with trastuzumab followed by adjuvant trastuzumab versus neoadjuvant chemotherapy alone, in patients with HER2-positive locally advanced breast cancer (the NOAH trial): a randomised controlled superiority trial with a parallel HER2-negative cohort. *Lancet*, 2010, 375(9712), 377-384.

[23] Kim, MM; Allen, P; Gonzalez-Angulo, AM; Woodward, WA; Meric-Bernstam, F; Buzdar, AU; et al. Pathologic complete response to neoadjuvant chemotherapy with trastuzumab predicts improved survival in women with HER2-overexpressing breast cancer. *Ann. Oncol.*, 2013, 24(8), 1999-2004.

[24] Huober, J; von, MG; Denkert, C; Tesch, H; Weiss, E; Zahm, DM; et al. Effect of neoadjuvant anthracycline-taxane-based chemotherapy in different biological breast cancer phenotypes: overall results from the GeparTrio study. *Breast Cancer Res. Treat.*, 2010, 124(1), 133-140.

[25] Senkus, E; Kyriakides, S; Penault-Llorca, F; Poortmans, P; Thompson, A; Zackrisson, S; et al. Primary breast cancer: ESMO Clinical Practice Guidelines for diagnosis, treatment and follow-up. *Ann. Oncol.*, 2013, 24 Suppl 6vi7-23.

[26] "Breast Cancer NCCN Guidelines Version 3.2013." *National Comprehensive Cancer Network*, 03 Aug. 2013. Web. 17 Nov. 2013.

[27] Roila, F; Boschetti, E; Tonato, M; Basurto, C; Bracarda, S; Picciafuoco, M; et al. Predictive factors of delayed emesis in cisplatin-treated patients and antiemetic activity and tolerability of metoclopramide or dexamethasone. A randomized single-blind study. *Am. J. Clin. Oncol.*, 1991, 14(3), 238-242.

[28] Kris, MG; Gralla, RJ; Clark, RA; Tyson, LB; O'Connell, JP; Wertheim, MS; et al. Incidence, course, and severity of delayed nausea and vomiting following the administration of high-dose cisplatin. *J. Clin. Oncol.*, 1985, 3(10), 1379-1384.

[29] Roila, F; Donati, D; Tamberi, S; Margutti, G. Delayed emesis: incidence, pattern, prognostic factors and optimal treatment. *Support. Care Cancer*, 2002, 10(2), 88-95.

[30] Morrow, GR; Roscoe, JA; Kirshner, JJ; Hynes, HE; Rosenbluth, RJ. Anticipatory nausea and vomiting in the era of 5-HT3 antiemetics. *Support. Care Cancer*, 1998, 6(3), 244-247.

[31] Andrews, PL; Davis, CJ; Bingham, S; Davidson, HI; Hawthorn, J; Maskell, L. The abdominal visceral innervation and the emetic reflex: pathways, pharmacology, and plasticity. *Can. J. Physiol Pharmacol.*, 1990, 68(2), 325-345.

[32] Higgins, GA; Kilpatrick, GJ; Bunce, KT; Jones, BJ; Tyers, MB. 5-HT3 receptor antagonists injected into the area postrema inhibit cisplatin-induced emesis in the ferret. *Br. J. Pharmacol.*, 1989, 97(1), 247-255.

[33] Carpenter, DO; Briggs, DB; Strominger, N. Responses of neurons of canine area postrema to neurotransmitters and peptides. *Cell Mol. Neurobiol.*, 1983, 3(2), 113-126.

[34] Wang, SC; Borison, HL. The vomiting center; a critical experimental analysis. *Arch. Neurol. Psychiatry*, 1950, 63(6), 928-941.

[35] Miller, AD; Wilson, VJ. 'Vomiting center' reanalyzed: an electrical stimulation study. *Brain Res.*, 1983, 270(1), 154-158.

[36] Sanger, GJ; Andrews, PL. Treatment of nausea and vomiting: gaps in our knowledge. *Auton. Neurosci.*, 2006, 129(1-2), 3-16.

[37] Zagon, A; Totterdell, S; Jones, RS. Direct projections from the ventrolateral medulla oblongata to the limbic forebrain: anterograde and retrograde tract-tracing studies in the rat. *J. Comp Neurol.*, 1994, 340(4), 445-468.

[38] Horn, CC; Ciucci, M; Chaudhury, A. Brain Fos expression during 48 h after cisplatin treatment: neural pathways for acute and delayed visceral sickness. *Auton. Neurosci.*, 2007, 132(1-2), 44-51.

[39] Saller, R; Hellenbrecht, D. High doses of metoclopramide or droperidol in the prevention of cisplatin-induced emesis. *Eur. J. Cancer Clin. Oncol.*, 1986, 22(10), 1199-1203.

[40] Endo, T; Minami, M; Hirafuji, M; Ogawa, T; Akita, K; Nemoto, M; et al. Neurochemistry and neuropharmacology of emesis - the role of serotonin. *Toxicology*, 2000, 153(1-3), 189-201.

[41] Fukui, H; Yamamoto, M; Sato, S. Vagal afferent fibers and peripheral 5-HT3 receptors mediate cisplatin-induced emesis in dogs. *Jpn. J. Pharmacol.*, 1992, 59(2), 221-226.

[42] Miner, WD; Sanger, GJ; Turner, DH. Evidence that 5-hydroxytryptamine3 receptors mediate cytotoxic drug and radiation-evoked emesis. *Br. J. Cancer*, 1987, 56(2), 159-162.
[43] Saito, R; Takano, Y; Kamiya, HO. Roles of substance P and NK(1) receptor in the brainstem in the development of emesis. *J. Pharmacol. Sci.*, 2003, 91(2), 87-94.
[44] Severini, C; Improta, G; Falconieri-Erspamer, G; Salvadori, S; Erspamer, V. The tachykinin peptide family. *Pharmacol. Rev.*, 2002, 54(2), 285-322.
[45] Quartara, L; Maggi, CA. The tachykinin NK1 receptor. Part II: Distribution and pathophysiological roles. *Neuropeptides*, 1998, 32(1), 1-49.
[46] Tattersall, FD; Rycroft, W; Francis, B; Pearce, D; Merchant, K; MacLeod, AM; et al. Tachykinin NK1 receptor antagonists act centrally to inhibit emesis induced by the chemotherapeutic agent cisplatin in ferrets. *Neuropharmacology*, 1996, 35(8), 1121-1129.
[47] Hesketh, PJ; Van, BS; Aapro, M; Tattersall, FD; Naylor, RJ; Hargreaves, R; et al. Differential involvement of neurotransmitters through the time course of cisplatin-induced emesis as revealed by therapy with specific receptor antagonists. *Eur. J. Cancer*, 2003, 39(8), 1074-1080.
[48] Roila, F; Herrstedt, J; Aapro, M; Gralla, RJ; Einhorn, LH; Ballatori, E; et al. Guideline update for MASCC and ESMO in the prevention of chemotherapy- and radiotherapy-induced nausea and vomiting: results of the Perugia consensus conference. *Ann. Oncol.*, 2010, 21 Suppl 5v232-v243.
[49] Feyer, P; Jordan, K. Update and new trends in antiemetic therapy: the continuing need for novel therapies. *Ann. Oncol.*, 2011, 22(1), 30-38.
[50] "MASCC/ESMO Antiemetic Guideline 2013." *Multinational Association of Supportive Care in Cancer,* 2013, Web. 17 Nov. 2013.
[51] Herrstedt, J; Rapoport, B; Warr, D; Roila, F; Bria, E; Rittenberg, C; et al. Acute emesis: moderately emetogenic chemotherapy. *Support. Care Cancer*, 2011, 19 Suppl 1S15-S23.
[52] Basch, E; Prestrud, AA; Hesketh, PJ; Kris, MG; Feyer, PC; Somerfield, MR; et al. Antiemetics: American Society of Clinical Oncology clinical practice guideline update. *J. Clin. Oncol.*, 2011, 29(31), 4189-4198.
[53] "Antiemesis NCCN Guidelines Version I.2014." *National Comprehensive Cancer Network*, 19 Aug. 2013. Web. 17, Nov. 2013.

[54] Hesketh, PJ; Kris, MG; Grunberg, SM; Beck, T; Hainsworth, JD; Harker, G; et al. Proposal for classifying the acute emetogenicity of cancer chemotherapy. *J. Clin. Oncol.*, 1997, 15(1), 103-109.

[55] Botrel, TE; Clark, OA; Clark, L; Paladini, L; Faleiros, E; Pegoretti, B. Efficacy of palonosetron (PAL) compared to other serotonin inhibitors (5-HT3R) in preventing chemotherapy-induced nausea and vomiting (CINV) in patients receiving moderately or highly emetogenic (MoHE) treatment: systematic review and meta-analysis. *Support. Care Cancer*, 2011, 19(6), 823-832.

[56] Warr, DG; Hesketh, PJ; Gralla, RJ; Muss, HB; Herrstedt, J; Eisenberg, PD; et al. Efficacy and tolerability of aprepitant for the prevention of chemotherapy-induced nausea and vomiting in patients with breast cancer after moderately emetogenic chemotherapy. *J. Clin. Oncol.*, 2005 23(12), 2822-2830.

[57] Grunberg, SM; Dugan, M; Muss, H; Wood, M; Burdette-Radoux, S; Weisberg, T; et al. Effectiveness of a single-day three-drug regimen of dexamethasone, palonosetron, and aprepitant for the prevention of acute and delayed nausea and vomiting caused by moderately emetogenic chemotherapy. *Support. Care Cancer*, 2009, 17(5), 589-594.

[58] Gralla, R; Bosnjak, S; Balser, C; Rizzi, G; Borroni, M; Rossi, G; et al. Prevention of chemotherapy induced nausea and vomiting (CINV) over repeated chemotherapy cyclies: results of a phase 3 trial of NEPA, a fixed oral dose combination of netupitant and palonosetron. *Eur. J. Cancer*, 2013, 49(supplement 2), s267-

[59] Grunberg, SM. Chemotherapy-induced nausea and vomiting: prevention, detection, and treatment--how are we doing? *J. Support. Oncol.*, 2004, 2(1 Suppl 1), 1-10, inside.

[60] Olson, RD; Mushlin, PS. Doxorubicin cardiotoxicity: analysis of prevailing hypotheses. *FASEB J.*, 1990, 4(13), 3076-3086.

[61] Zweier, JL; Gianni, L; Muindi, J; Myers, CE. Differences in O2 reduction by the iron complexes of adriamycin and daunomycin: the importance of the sidechain hydroxyl group. *Biochim. Biophys. Acta*, 1986, 884(2), 326-336.

[62] Powis, G. Free radical formation by antitumor quinones. *Free Radic. Biol. Med.*, 1989, 6(1), 63-101.

[63] Trush, MA; Kensler, TW. An overview of the relationship between oxidative stress and chemical carcinogenesis. *Free Radic. Biol. Med.*, 1991, 10(3-4), 201-209.

[64] Griffin-Green, EA; Zaleska, MM; Erecinska, M. Adriamycin-induced lipid peroxidation in mitochondria and microsomes. *Biochem. Pharmacol.*, 1988, 37(16), 3071-3077.
[65] Hasinoff, BB; Davey, JP. Adriamycin and its iron(III) and copper(II) complexes. Glutathione-induced dissociation; cytochrome c oxidase inactivation and protection; binding to cardiolipin. *Biochem. Pharmacol.*, 1988, 37(19), 3663-3669.
[66] Esterbauer, H; Zollner, H. Methods for determination of aldehydic lipid peroxidation products. *Free Radic. Biol. Med.*, 1989, 7(2), 197-203.
[67] Esterbauer, H; Schaur, RJ; Zollner, H. Chemistry and biochemistry of 4-hydroxynonenal, malonaldehyde and related aldehydes. *Free Radic. Biol. Med.*, 1991, 11(1), 81-128.
[68] Loidl-Stahlhofen, A; Spiteller, G. alpha-Hydroxyaldehydes, products of lipid peroxidation. *Biochim. Biophys. Acta*, 1994, 1211(2), 156-160.
[69] Witz, G. Biological interactions of alpha,beta-unsaturated aldehydes. *Free Radic. Biol. Med.*, 1989, 7(3), 333-349.
[70] Luo, X; Evrovsky, Y; Cole, D; Trines, J; Benson, LN; Lehotay, DC. Doxorubicin-induced acute changes in cytotoxic aldehydes, antioxidant status and cardiac function in the rat. *Biochim. Biophys. Acta*, 1997, 1360(1), 45-52.
[71] Doroshow, JH. Effect of anthracycline antibiotics on oxygen radical formation in rat heart. *Cancer Res.*, 1983, 43(2), 460-472.
[72] Ryan, TP; Aust, SD. The role of iron in oxygen-mediated toxicities. *Crit Rev. Toxicol.*, 1992, 22(2), 119-141.
[73] Minotti, G. Sources and role of iron in lipid peroxidation. *Chem. Res. Toxicol.*, 1993, 6(2), 134-146.
[74] Mimnaugh, EG; Siddik, ZH; Drew, R; Sikic, BI; Gram, TE. The effects of alpha-tocopherol on the toxicity, disposition, and metabolism of adriamycin in mice. *Toxicol. Appl. Pharmacol.*, 1979, 49(1), 119-126.
[75] Doroshow, JH; Locker, GY; Ifrim, I; Myers, CE. Prevention of doxorubicin cardiac toxicity in the mouse by N-acetylcysteine. *J. Clin. Invest*, 1981, 68(4), 1053-1064.
[76] Myers, C; Bonow, R; Palmeri, S; Jenkins, J; Corden, B; Locker, G; et al. A randomized controlled trial assessing the prevention of doxorubicin cardiomyopathy by N-acetylcysteine. *Semin. Oncol.*, 1983, 10(1 Suppl 1), 53-55.
[77] Minotti, G; Mancuso, C; Frustaci, A; Mordente, A; Santini, SA; Calafiore, AM; et al. Paradoxical inhibition of cardiac lipid peroxidation in cancer patients treated with doxorubicin. Pharmacologic and

molecular reappraisal of anthracycline cardiotoxicity. *J. Clin. Invest*, 1996, 98(3), 650-661.

[78] Talcott, RE; Smith, MT; Giannini, DD. Inhibition of microsomal lipid peroxidation by naphthoquinones: structure-activity relationships and possible mechanisms of action. *Arch. Biochem. Biophys.*, 1985, 241(1), 88-94.

[79] Kang, YJ; Chen, Y; Epstein, PN. Suppression of doxorubicin cardiotoxicity by overexpression of catalase in the heart of transgenic mice. *J. Biol. Chem.*, 1996, 271(21), 12610-12616.

[80] Jensen, RA. Doxorubicin cardiotoxicity: contractile changes after long-term treatment in the rat. *J. Pharmacol. Exp. Ther.*, 1986, 236(1), 197-203.

[81] Rabkin, SW. Interaction of external calcium concentration and verapamil on the effects of doxorubicin (adriamycin) in the isolated heart preparation. *J. Cardiovasc. Pharmacol.*, 1983, 5(5), 848-855.

[82] Revis, NW; Marusic, N. Effects of doxorubicin and its aglycone metabolite on calcium sequestration by rabbit heart, liver, and kidney mitochondria. *Life Sci.*, 1979, 25(12), 1055-1063.

[83] Bachmann, E; Zbinden, G. Effect of doxorubicin and rubidazone on respiratory function and Ca^{2+} transport in rat heart mitochondria. *Toxicology Letters*, 1979, 3(1), 29-34.

[84] Solem, LE; Wallace, KB. Selective activation of the sodium-independent, cyclosporin A-sensitive calcium pore of cardiac mitochondria by doxorubicin. *Toxicol. Appl. Pharmacol.*, 1993, 121(1), 50-57.

[85] Singal, PK; Deally, CM; Weinberg, LE. Subcellular effects of adriamycin in the heart: a concise review. *J. Mol. Cell Cardiol.*, 1987, 19(8), 817-828.

[86] Ferrero, ME; Ferrero, E; Gaja, G; Bernelli-Zazzera, A. Adriamycin: energy metabolism and mitochondrial oxidations in the heart of treated rabbits. *Biochem. Pharmacol.*, 1976, 25(2), 125-130.

[87] Iwamoto, Y; Hansen, IL; Porter, TH; Folkers, K. Inhibition of coenzyme Q10-enzymes, succinoxidase and NADH-oxidase, by adriamycin and other quinones having antitumor activity. *Biochem. Biophys. Res. Commun.*, 1974, 58(3), 633-638.

[88] Gosalvez, M; Blanco, M; Hunter, J; Miko, M; Chance, B. Effects of anticancer agents on the respiration of isolated mitochondria and tumor cells. *Eur. J. Cancer*, 1974, 10(9), 567-574.

[89] Lefrak, EA; Pitha, J; Rosenheim, S; Gottlieb, JA. A clinicopathologic analysis of adriamycin cardiotoxicity. *Cancer*, 1973, 32(2), 302-314.

[90] Meredith, MJ; Reed, DJ. Depletion in vitro of mitochondrial glutathione in rat hepatocytes and enhancement of lipid peroxidation by adriamycin and1,3-bis(2-chloroethyl)-1-nitrosourea(BCNU).*Biochem. Pharmacol.*, 1983, 32(8), 1383-1388.

[91] Duarte-Karim, M; Ruysschaert, JM; Hildebrand, J. Affinity of adriamycin to phospholipids. A possible explanation for cardiac mitochondrial lesions. *Biochem. Biophys. Res. Commun.*, 1976, 71(2), 658-663.

[92] Ardail, D; Privat, JP; Egret-Charlier, M; Levrat, C; Lerme, F; Louisot, P. Mitochondrial contact sites. Lipid composition and dynamics. *J. Biol. Chem.*, 1990, 265(31), 18797-18802.

[93] Schlame, M; Rua, D; Greenberg, ML. The biosynthesis and functional role of cardiolipin. *Prog. Lipid Res.*, 2000, 39(3), 257-288.

[94] Goormaghtigh, E; Huart, P; Praet, M; Brasseur, R; Ruysschaert, JM. Structure of the adriamycin-cardiolipin complex. Role in mitochondrial toxicity. *Biophys. Chem.*, 1990, 35(2-3), 247-257.

[95] Goormaghtigh, E; Chatelain, P; Caspers, J; Ruysschaert, JM. Evidence of a complex between adriamycin derivatives and cardiolipin: possible role in cardiotoxicity. *Biochem. Pharmacol.*, 1980, 29(21), 3003-3010.

[96] Davies, KJ; Doroshow, JH; Hochstein, P. Mitochondrial NADH dehydrogenase-catalyzed oxygen radical production by adriamycin, and the relative inactivity of 5-iminodaunorubicin. *FEBS Lett.*, 1983, 153(1), 227-230.

[97] Davies, KJ; Doroshow, JH. Redox cycling of anthracyclines by cardiac mitochondria. I. Anthracycline radical formation by NADH dehydrogenase. *J. Biol. Chem.*, 1986, 261(7), 3060-3067.

[98] Doroshow, JH; Davies, KJ. Redox cycling of anthracyclines by cardiac mitochondria. II. Formation of superoxide anion, hydrogen peroxide, and hydroxyl radical. *J. Biol. Chem.*, 1986, 261(7), 3068-3074.

[99] Zhou, S; Palmeira, CM; Wallace, KB. Doxorubicin-induced persistent oxidative stress to cardiac myocytes. *Toxicol. Lett.*, 2001, 121(3), 151-157.

[100] Minotti, G; Cavaliere, AF; Mordente, A; Rossi, M; Schiavello, R; Zamparelli, R; et al. Secondary alcohol metabolites mediate iron delocalization in cytosolic fractions of myocardial biopsies exposed to anticancer anthracyclines. Novel linkage between anthracycline

metabolism and iron-induced cardiotoxicity. *J. Clin. Invest*, 1995, 95(4), 1595-1605.

[101] Del, TM; Danesi, R; Ducci, M; Bernardini, C; Romanini, A. Might adriamycinol contribute to adriamycin-induced cardiotoxicity? *Pharmacol. Res. Commun.*, 1985, 17(11), 1073-1084.

[102] Olson, RD; Mushlin, PS; Brenner, DE; Fleischer, S; Cusack, BJ; Chang, BK; et al. Doxorubicin cardiotoxicity may be caused by its metabolite, doxorubicinol. *Proc. Natl. Acad. Sci. U. S. A*, 1988, 85(10), 3585-3589.

[103] Boucek, RJ, Jr.; Olson, RD; Brenner, DE; Ogunbunmi, EM; Inui, M; Fleischer, S. The major metabolite of doxorubicin is a potent inhibitor of membrane-associated ion pumps. A correlative study of cardiac muscle with isolated membrane fractions. *J. Biol. Chem.*, 1987, 262(33), 15851-15856.

[104] Minotti, G; Recalcati, S; Mordente, A; Liberi, G; Calafiore, AM; Mancuso, C; et al. The secondary alcohol metabolite of doxorubicin irreversibly inactivates aconitase/iron regulatory protein-1 in cytosolic fractions from human myocardium. *FASEB J.*, 1998, 12(7), 541-552.

[105] Bachur, NR; Gee, MV; Friedman, RD. Nuclear catalyzed antibiotic free radical formation. *Cancer Res.*, 1982, 42(3), 1078-1081.

[106] Keizer, HG; Pinedo, HM; Schuurhuis, GJ; Joenje, H. Doxorubicin (adriamycin): a critical review of free radical-dependent mechanisms of cytotoxicity. *Pharmacol. Ther.*, 1990, 47(2), 219-231.

[107] Jeyaseelan, R; Poizat, C; Wu, HY; Kedes, L. Molecular mechanisms of doxorubicin-induced cardiomyopathy. Selective suppression of Reiske iron-sulfur protein, ADP/ATP translocase, and phosphofructokinase genes is associated with ATP depletion in rat cardiomyocytes. *J. Biol. Chem.*, 1997, 272(9), 5828-5832.

[108] Kurabayashi, M; Jeyaseelan, R; Kedes, L. Antineoplastic agent doxorubicin inhibits myogenic differentiation of C2 myoblasts. *J. Biol. Chem.*, 1993, 268(8), 5524-5529.

[109] Kurabayashi, M; Dutta, S; Jeyaseelan, R; Kedes, L. Doxorubicin-induced Id2A gene transcription is targeted at an activating transcription factor/cyclic AMP response element motif through novel mechanisms involving protein kinases distinct from protein kinase C and protein kinase A. *Mol. Cell Biol.*, 1995, 15(11), 6386-6397.

[110] Arai, M; Tomaru, K; Takizawa, T; Sekiguchi, K; Yokoyama, T; Suzuki, T; et al. Sarcoplasmic reticulum genes are selectively down-regul in cardiomyopathy produced by doxorubicin in rabbits. *J. Mol. Cell Cardiol.*, 1998, 30(2), 243-254.

[111] Tomlinson, CW; McGrath, GM; McNeill, JH. Adriamycin cardiomyopathy: pathological and membrane functional changes in a canine model with mild impairment of left ventricular function. *Can. J. Cardiol.*, 1986, 2(6), 368-374.

[112] Ito, H; Miller, SC; Billingham, ME; Akimoto, H; Torti, SV; Wade, R; et al. Doxorubicin selectively inhibits muscle gene expression in cardiac muscle cells in vivo and in vitro. *Proc. Natl. Acad. Sci. U. S. A*, 1990, 87(11), 4275-4279.

[113] Zheng, Z; Pavlidis, P; Chua, S; D'Agati, VD; Gharavi, AG. An ancestral haplotype defines susceptibility to doxorubicin nephropathy in the laboratory mouse. *J. Am. Soc. Nephrol.*, 2006, 17(7), 1796-1800.

[114] Anderson, AB; Arriaga, EA. Subcellular metabolite profiles of the parent CCRF-CEM and the derived CEM/C2 cell lines after treatment with doxorubicin. *J. Chromatogr. B Analyt. Technol. Biomed. Life Sci.*, 2004, 808(2), 295-302.

[115] Tokarska-Schlattner, M; Zaugg, M; da, SR; Lucchinetti, E; Schaub, MC; Wallimann, T; et al. Acute toxicity of doxorubicin on isolated perfused heart: response of kinases regulating energy supply. *Am. J. Physiol Heart Circ. Physiol*, 2005, 289(1), H37-H47.

[116] Zagotto, G; Gatto, B; Moro, S; Sissi, C; Palumbo, M. Anthracyclines: recent developments in their separation and quantitation. *J. Chromatogr. B Biomed. Sci. Appl.*, 2001, 764(1-2), 161-171.

[117] van, AJ; van, TO; Tijssen, F; Schinkel, AH; Beijnen, JH. Increased accumulation of doxorubicin and doxorubicinol in cardiac tissue of mice lacking mdr1a P-glycoprotein. *Br. J. Cancer*, 1999, 79(1), 108-113.

[118] Stewart, DJ; Grewaal, D; Green, RM; Mikhael, N; Goel, R; Montpetit, VA; et al. Concentrations of doxorubicin and its metabolites in human autopsy heart and other tissues. *Anticancer Res.*, 1993, 13(6A), 1945-1952.

[119] Curigliano, G; Cardinale, D; Suter, T; Plataniotis, G; de, AE; Sandri, MT; et al. Cardiovascular toxicity induced by chemotherapy, targeted agents and radiotherapy: ESMO Clinical Practice Guidelines. *Ann. Oncol.*, 2012, 23 Suppl 7vii155-vii166.

[120] Doroshow, JH. Doxorubicin-induced cardiac toxicity. *N. Engl. J. Med.*, 1991, 324(12), 843-845.

[121] Wortman, JE; Lucas, VS, Jr.; Schuster, E; Thiele, D; Logue, GL. Sudden death during doxorubicin administration. *Cancer*, 1979, 44(5), 1588-1591.

[122] Olson, HM; Young, DM; Prieur, DJ; LeRoy, AF; Reagan, RL. Electrolyte and morphologic alterations of myocardium in adriamycin-treated rabbits. *Am. J. Pathol.*, 1974, 77(3), 439-454.

[123] Iwasaki, T; Suzuki, T. Ultrastructural alterations of the myocardium induced by doxorubicin. A scanning electron microscopic study. *Virchows Arch. B Cell Pathol. Incl. Mol. Pathol.*, 1991, 60(1), 35-39.

[124] Mettler, FP; Young, DM; Ward, JM. Adriamycin-induced cardiotoxicity (cardiomyopathy and congestive heart failure) in rats. *Cancer Res.*, 1977, 37(8 Pt 1), 2705-2713.

[125] Von Hoff, DD; Layard, MW; Basa, P; Davis, HL, Jr.; Von Hoff, AL; Rozencweig, M; et al. Risk factors for doxorubicin-induced congestive heart failure. *Ann. Intern. Med.*, 1979, 91(5), 710-717.

[126] Steinherz, LJ; Steinherz, PG; Tan, CT; Heller, G; Murphy, ML. Cardiac toxicity 4 to 20 years after completing anthracycline therapy. *JAMA*, 1991, 266(12), 1672-1677.

[127] Legha, SS; Benjamin, RS; Mackay, B; Ewer, M; Wallace, S; Valdivieso, M; et al. Reduction of doxorubicin cardiotoxicity by prolonged continuous intravenous infusion. *Ann. Intern. Med.*, 1982, 96(2), 133-139.

[128] Danesi, R; Fogli, S; Gennari, A; Conte, P; Del, TM. Pharmacokinetic-pharmacodynamic relationships of the anthracycline anticancer drugs. *Clin. Pharmacokinet.*, 2002, 41(6), 431-444.

[129] Cusack, BJ; Young, SP; Driskell, J; Olson, RD. Doxorubicin and doxorubicinol pharmacokinetics and tissue concentrations following bolus injection and continuous infusion of doxorubicin in the rabbit. *Cancer Chemother. Pharmacol.*, 1993, 32(1), 53-58.

[130] Fidler, IJ; Barnes, Z; Fogler, WE; Kirsh, R; Bugelski, P; Poste, G. Involvement of macrophages in the eradication of established metastases following intravenous injection of liposomes containing macrophage activators. *Cancer Res.*, 1982, 42(2), 496-501.

[131] Plosker, GL. Pegylated liposomal Doxorubicin: a review of its use in the treatment of relapsed or refractory multiple myeloma. *Drugs*, 2008, 68(17), 2535-2551.

[132] Vail, DM; Amantea, MA; Colbern, GT; Martin, FJ; Hilger, RA; Working, PK. Pegylated liposomal doxorubicin: proof of principle using preclinical animal models and pharmacokinetic studies. *Semin. Oncol.*, 2004, 31(6 Suppl 13), 16-35.

[133] Hanahan, D; Bergers, G; Bergsland, E. Less is more, regularly: metronomic dosing of cytotoxic drugs can target tumor angiogenesis in mice. *J. Clin. Invest*, 2000, 105(8), 1045-1047.

[134] Sun, K; Wang, J; Zhang, J; Hua, M; Liu, C; Chen, T. Dextran-g-PEI nanoparticles as a carrier for co-delivery of adriamycin and plasmid into osteosarcoma cells. *Int. J. Biol. Macromol.*, 2011, 49(2), 173-180.

[135] Singal, PK; Iliskovic, N. Doxorubicin-induced cardiomyopathy. *N. Engl. J. Med.*, 1998, 339(13), 900-905.

[136] Singal, PK; Li, T; Kumar, D; Danelisen, I; Iliskovic, N. Adriamycin-induced heart failure: mechanism and modulation. *Mol. Cell Biochem.*, 2000, 207(1-2), 77-86.

[137] Singal, PK; Iliskovic, N; Li, T; Kumar, D. Adriamycin cardiomyopathy: pathophysiology and prevention. *FASEB J.*, 1997, 11(12), 931-936.

[138] Minotti, G; Cairo, G; Monti, E. Role of iron in anthracycline cardiotoxicity: new tunes for an old song? *FASEB J.*, 1999, 13(2), 199-212.

[139] Zucchi, R; Danesi, R. Cardiac toxicity of antineoplastic anthracyclines. *Curr. Med. Chem. Anticancer Agents*, 2003, 3(2), 151-171.

[140] Ladas, EJ; Jacobson, JS; Kennedy, DD; Teel, K; Fleischauer, A; Kelly, KM. Antioxidants and cancer therapy: a systematic review. *J. Clin. Oncol.*, 2004, 22(3), 517-528.

[141] Dorr, RT. Cytoprotective agents for anthracyclines. *Semin. Oncol.*, 1996, 23(4 Suppl 8), 23-34.

[142] Yuhas, JM. Active versus passive absorption kinetics as the basis for selective protection of normal tissues by S-2-(3-aminopropylamino)-ethylphosphorothioic acid. *Cancer Res.*, 1980, 40(5), 1519-1524.

[143] Dorr, RT; Lagel, K; McLean, S. Cardioprotection of rat heart myocytes with amifostine (Ethyol) and its free thiol, WR-1065, in vitro. *Eur. J. Cancer*, 1996, 32A Suppl 4S21-S25.

[144] Nazeyrollas, P; Prevost, A; Baccard, N; Manot, L; Devillier, P; Millart, H. Effects of amifostine on perfused isolated rat heart and on acute doxorubicin-induced cardiotoxicity. *Cancer Chemother. Pharmacol.*, 1999, 43(3), 227-232.

[145] Yurekli, Y; Unak, P; Ertay, T; Biber, Z; Medine, I; Teksoz, S. Radiopharmaceutical model using 99mTc-MIBI to evaluate amifostine protection against doxorubicin cardiotoxicity in rats. *Ann. Nucl. Med.*, 2005, 19(3), 197-200.

[146] Bolaman, Z; Cicek, C; Kadikoylu, G; Barutca, S; Serter, M; Yenisey, C; et al. The protective effects of amifostine on adriamycin-induced acute cardiotoxicity in rats. *Tohoku J. Exp. Med.*, 2005, 207(4), 249-253.

[147] Nazeyrollas, P; Frances, C; Prevost, A; Costa, B; Lorenzato, M; Kantelip, JP; et al. Efficiency of amifostine as a protection against doxorubicin toxicity in rats during a 12-day treatment. *Anticancer Res.*, 2003, 23(1A), 405-409.

[148] Rigatos, SK; Stathopoulos, GP; Dontas, I; Perrea-Kotsarelis, D; Couris, E; Karayannacos, PE; et al. Investigation of doxorubicin tissue toxicity: does amifostine provide chemoprotection? An experimental study. *Anticancer Res.*, 2002, 22(1A), 129-134.

[149] Jahnukainen, K; Jahnukainen, T; Salmi, TT; Svechnikov, K; Eksborg, S; Soder, O. Amifostine protects against early but not late toxic effects of doxorubicin in infant rats. *Cancer Res.*, 2001, 61(17), 6423-6427.

[150] Catino, A; Crucitta, E; Latorre, A; Sambiasi, D; Calabrese, P; Lorusso, V. Amifostine as chemoprotectant in metastatic breast cancer patients treated with doxorubicin. *Oncol. Rep.*, 2003, 10(1), 163-167.

[151] Spath-Schwalbe, E; Lange, C; Genvresse, I; Kruger, L; Eucker, J; Schweigert, M; et al. Influence of amifostine on toxicity of CHOP in elderly patients with aggressive non-Hodgkin's lymphoma--a phase II study. *Anticancer Drugs*, 2002, 13(4), 395-403.

[152] Creighton, AM; Birnie, GD. The effect of bisdioxopiperazines on the synthesis of deoxyribonucleic acid, ribonucleic acid and protein in growing mouse-embryo fibroblasts. *Biochem. J.*, 1969, 114(4), 58P-

[153] Schroeder, PE; Davidson, JN; Hasinoff, BB. Dihydroorotase catalyzes the ring opening of the hydrolysis intermediates of the cardioprotective drug dexrazoxane (ICRF-187). *Drug Metab Dispos.*, 2002, 30(12), 1431-1435.

[154] Hasinoff, BB; Schnabl, KL; Marusak, RA; Patel, D; Huebner, E. Dexrazoxane (ICRF-187) protects cardiac myocytes against doxorubicin by preventing damage to mitochondria. *Cardiovasc. Toxicol.*, 2003, 3(2), 89-99.

[155] Hasinoff, BB; Schroeder, PE; Patel, D. The metabolites of the cardioprotective drug dexrazoxane do not protect myocytes from doxorubicin-induced cytotoxicity. *Mol. Pharmacol.*, 2003, 64(3), 670-678.

[156] Junjing, Z; Yan, Z; Baolu, Z. Scavenging effects of dexrazoxane on free radicals. *J. Clin. Biochem. Nutr.*, 2010, 47(3), 238-245.

[157] Rajagopalan, S; Politi, PM; Sinha, BK; Myers, CE. Adriamycin-induced free radical formation in the perfused rat heart: implications for cardiotoxicity. *Cancer Res.*, 1988, 48(17), 4766-4769.

[158] Popelova, O; Sterba, M; Haskova, P; Simunek, T; Hroch, M; Guncova, I; et al. Dexrazoxane-afforded protection against chronic anthracycline cardiotoxicity in vivo: effective rescue of cardiomyocytes from apoptotic cell death. *Br. J. Cancer*, 2009, 101(5), 792-802.

[159] Sargent, JM; Williamson, CJ; Yardley, C; Taylor, CG; Hellmann, K. Dexrazoxane significantly impairs the induction of doxorubicin resistance in the human leukaemia line, K562. *Br. J. Cancer*, 2001, 84(7), 959-964.

[160] Bjelogrlic, SK; Radic, J; Radulovic, S; Jokanovic, M; Jovic, V. Effects of dexrazoxane and amifostine on evolution of Doxorubicin cardiomyopathy in vivo. *Exp. Biol. Med. (Maywood.)*, 2007, 232(11), 1414-1424.

[161] Bjelogrlic, SK; Lukic, ST; Djuricic, SM. Activity of dexrazoxane and amifostine against late cardiotoxicity induced by the combination of doxorubicin and cyclophosphamide in vivo. *Basic Clin. Pharmacol. Toxicol.*, 2013, 113(4), 228-238.

[162] Speyer, JL; Green, MD; Zeleniuch-Jacquotte, A; Wernz, JC; Rey, M; Sanger, J; et al. ICRF-187 permits longer treatment with doxorubicin in women with breast cancer. *J. Clin. Oncol.*, 1992, 10(1), 117-127.

[163] Speyer, JL; Green, MD; Kramer, E; Rey, M; Sanger, J; Ward, C; et al. Protective effect of the bispiperazinedione ICRF-187 against doxorubicin-induced cardiac toxicity in women with advanced breast cancer. *N. Engl. J. Med.*, 1988, 319(12), 745-752.

[164] Swain, SM; Whaley, FS; Gerber, MC; Weisberg, S; York, M; Spicer, D; et al. Cardioprotection with dexrazoxane for doxorubicin-containing therapy in advanced breast cancer. *J. Clin. Oncol.*, 1997, 15(4), 1318-1332.

[165] Marty, M; Espie, M; Llombart, A; Monnier, A; Rapoport, BL; Stahalova, V. Multicenter randomized phase III study of the cardioprotective effect of dexrazoxane (Cardioxane) in advanced/metastatic breast cancer patients treated with anthracycline-based chemotherapy. *Ann. Oncol.*, 2006, 17(4), 614-622.

[166] Lipshultz, SE; Rifai, N; Dalton, VM; Levy, DE; Silverman, LB; Lipsitz, SR; et al. The effect of dexrazoxane on myocardial injury in doxorubicin-treated children with acute lymphoblastic leukemia. *N. Engl. J. Med.*, 2004, 351(2), 145-153.

[167] Wexler, LH; Andrich, MP; Venzon, D; Berg, SL; Weaver-McClure, L; Chen, CC; et al. Randomized trial of the cardioprotective agent ICRF-187 in pediatric sarcoma patients treated with doxorubicin. *J. Clin. Oncol.*, 1996, 14(2), 362-372.

[168] Swain, SM; Whaley, FS; Gerber, MC; Ewer, MS; Bianchine, JR; Gams, RA. Delayed administration of dexrazoxane provides cardioprotection for patients with advanced breast cancer treated with doxorubicin-containing therapy. *J. Clin. Oncol.*, 1997, 15(4), 1333-1340.

[169] Verhoef, V; Filppi, J. Effect of the cardioprotective agent Adr-529 (Icrf-187) on the antitumor-activity of doxorubicin. *Proceedings of the American Association for Cancer Research*, 1988, 29

[170] Seymour, L; Bramwell, V; Moran, LA. Use of dexrazoxane as a cardioprotectant in patients receiving doxorubicin or epirubicin chemotherapy for the treatment of cancer. The Provincial Systemic Treatment Disease Site Group. *Cancer Prev. Control*, 1999, 3(2), 145-159.

[171] "Dexrazoxane: Official FDA information, side effects and uses." *Drugs*, Sep. 2012. Web. 19 Nov. 2013.

[172] Tebbi, CK; London, WB; Friedman, D; Villaluna, D; De Alarcon, PA; Constine, LS; et al. Dexrazoxane-associated risk for acute myeloid leukemia/myelodysplastic syndrome and other secondary malignancies in pediatric Hodgkin's disease. *J. Clin. Oncol.*, 2007, 25(5), 493-500.

[173] Salzer, WL; Devidas, M; Carroll, WL; Winick, N; Pullen, J; Hunger, SP; et al. Long-term results of the pediatric oncology group studies for childhood acute lymphoblastic leukemia 1984-2001: a report from the children's oncology group. *Leukemia*, 2010, 24(2), 355-370.

[174] Schwartz, CL; Constine, LS; Villaluna, D; London, WB; Hutchison, RE; Sposto, R; et al. A risk-adapted, response-based approach using ABVE-PC for children and adolescents with intermediate- and high-risk Hodgkin lymphoma: the results of P9425. *Blood*, 2009, 114(10), 2051-2059.

[175] "Dexrazoxane (Cardioxane): restriction of use to adults with advanced or metastatic breast cancer only." *Regulating Medicines and Medical Devices*, July 2011. Web. 19 Nov. 2013.

[176] Cardinale, D; Sandri, MT; Martinoni, A; Borghini, E; Civelli, M; Lamantia, G; et al. Myocardial injury revealed by plasma troponin I in breast cancer treated with high-dose chemotherapy. *Ann. Oncol.*, 2002, 13(5), 710-715.

[177] Cardinale, D; Sandri, MT; Colombo, A; Colombo, N; Boeri, M; Lamantia, G; et al. Prognostic value of troponin I in cardiac risk stratification of cancer patients undergoing high-dose chemotherapy. *Circulation*, 2004, 109(22), 2749-2754.

[178] Meinardi, MT; van Veldhuisen, DJ; Gietema, JA; Dolsma, WV; Boomsma, F; van den Berg, MP; et al. Prospective evaluation of early cardiac damage induced by epirubicin-containing adjuvant chemotherapy and locoregional radiotherapy in breast cancer patients. *J. Clin. Oncol.*, 2001, 19(10), 2746-2753.

[179] Nousiainen, T; Vanninen, E; Jantunen, E; Puustinen, J; Remes, J; Rantala, A; et al. Natriuretic peptides during the development of doxorubicin-induced left ventricular diastolic dysfunction. *J. Intern. Med.*, 2002, 251(3), 228-234.

[180] Zipes, DP; Camm, AJ; Borggrefe, M; Buxton, AE; Chaitman, B; Fromer, M; et al. ACC/AHA/ESC 2006 guidelines for management of patients with ventricular arrhythmias and the prevention of sudden cardiac death: a report of the American College of Cardiology/American Heart Association Task Force and the European Society of Cardiology Committee for Practice Guidelines (Writing Committee to Develop Guidelines for Management of Patients With Ventricular Arrhythmias and the Prevention of Sudden Cardiac Death). *J. Am. Coll. Cardiol.*, 2006, 48(5), e247-e346.

[181] Fuster, V; Ryden, LE; Cannom, DS; Crijns, HJ; Curtis, AB; Ellenbogen, KA; et al. ACC/AHA/ESC 2006 guidelines for the management of patients with atrial fibrillation: full text: a report of the American College of Cardiology/American Heart Association Task Force on practice guidelines and the European Society of Cardiology Committee for Practice Guidelines (Writing Committee to Revise the 2001 guidelines for the management of patients with atrial fibrillation) developed in collaboration with the European Heart Rhythm Association and the Heart Rhythm Society. *Europace.*, 2006, 8(9), 651-745.

[182] Rudzinski, T; Ciesielczyk, M; Religa, W; Bednarkiewicz, Z; Krzeminska-Pakula, M. Doxorubicin-induced ventricular arrhythmia treated by implantation of an automatic cardioverter-defibrillator. *Europace.*, 2007, 9(5), 278-280.

[183] McMurray, JJ; Adamopoulos, S; Anker, SD; Auricchio, A; Bohm, M; Dickstein, K; et al. ESC Guidelines for the diagnosis and treatment of acute and chronic heart failure 2012: The Task Force for the Diagnosis

and Treatment of Acute and Chronic Heart Failure 2012 of the European Society of Cardiology. Developed in collaboration with the Heart Failure Association (HFA) of the ESC. *Eur. Heart J.*, 2012, 33(14), 1787-1847.

[184] Cardinale, D; Colombo, A; Lamantia, G; Colombo, N; Civelli, M; De, GG; et al. Anthracycline-induced cardiomyopathy: clinical relevance and response to pharmacologic therapy. *J. Am. Coll. Cardiol.*, 2010, 55(3), 213-220.

[185] Ajijola, OA; Nandigam, KV; Chabner, BA; Orencole, M; Dec, GW; Ruskin, JN; et al. Usefulness of cardiac resynchronization therapy in the management of Doxorubicin-induced cardiomyopathy. *Am. J. Cardiol.*, 2008, 101(9), 1371-1372.

[186] Rickard, J; Kumbhani, DJ; Baranowski, B; Martin, DO; Tang, WH; Wilkoff, BL. Usefulness of cardiac resynchronization therapy in patients with Adriamycin-induced cardiomyopathy. *Am. J. Cardiol.*, 2010, 105(4), 522-526.

INDEX

A

D

E

F

G

K

L

M

N

O

P

Q

R

S

T

U

V

W

X

Y